● Skills for Practice ●

Statistics:

A Guide for Therapists

by

John McCall

BSc(Hons), MSc
Senior Lecturer, Department of Mathematical Sciences,
University of East London, UK

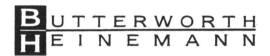

BUTTERWORTH
HEINEMANN

Butterworth-Heinemann
Linacre House, Jordan Hill, Oxford OX2 8DP
A division of Reed Educational and Professional Publishing Ltd

$\mathcal{R}$ A member of the Reed Elsevier plc group

OXFORD   BOSTON   JOHANNESBURG
MELBOURNE   NEW DELHI   SINGAPORE

First published 1996
© Reed Educational and Professional Publishing Ltd

British Library Cataloguing in Publication Data
A catalogue record for this book is available from the British Library.

Library of Congress Cataloguing in Publication Data
A catalogue record for this book is available from the Library of Congress.

ISBN 0 7506 2104 4

Printed and bound in Great Britain by Biddles Ltd, Guildford and Kings Lynn

Contents

Preface

This guide is designed to give an insight into the use of statistics in the treatment of data. It clearly cannot be a comprehensive treatise on the subject but, it is hoped, it will give an indication of the general nature of statistical procedures and will help the reader to understand more easily statistical arguments found in the literature and to become more confident when presenting the results of a research project, perhaps in a lecture or a publication.

Statistics of one kind or another are frequently provided by newspapers or other organizations and we can be forgiven, I think, if we gain the impression that 'you can prove anything with statistics.' The unwary may be taken in, if the intention is to deceive, and this is clearly not a recent concept. Consider the much quoted comment, attributed to Benjamin Disraeli, that 'there are lies, damned lies and statistics'.

Furthermore, for those who are unfamiliar with the subject, a comment such as 'half the children in this country are below average intelligence' may seem to be a cause for concern, whereas, by the very definition of the term (assuming that the spread of intelligence is symmetrical) this must be so. Also, it is unfortunate that the term 'average' is often considered to be almost synonymous with 'mediocre'. In magazines that are testing equipment, such as cameras, for the benefit of readers, one may read that the performance was 'only average' when the intention is to imply that it is not very good. It is strange that in such magazines virtually none of the equipment tested seems to be below average. Clearly such vague thinking has no place in the reporting of experimental work.

For anyone who is involved in conducting research, or who may be interested in the research of others, it is essential to have at least a basic knowledge of statistical procedures and to be clear about the meaning of the terms that are in common use. No measurement, when taken repeatedly, will have exactly the same result each time. This is a consequence of what is known as 'random error' which is an uncontrollable variability which will always be present, to a greater or lesser extent, no matter how carefully the measurements are taken. If such random errors did not exist, much of statistics would be unnecessary. However, having collected data, conclusions have to be drawn, in spite of such errors, and statistics will help in this process.

Consider also a situation where we may wish to collect values of some particular human function in order to determine the 'norm', for example lung capacity, grip strength or the number of words recognized by a child of six. These will clearly vary from one person to the next, so in order to consider the data in an ordered fashion, they need to be represented by a characteristic value, together with a measure of the way in which they vary between individuals. Once again, statistics comes to our aid.

One problem which may be encountered by therapists when conducting research is the comparison of a particular measurement between two groups of individuals, each having been given a different form of treatment. It is then required to decide whether the difference between the average value for each group represents a real difference or whether it simply results from the random variation mentioned above. Alternatively, the researcher may wish to determine whether a particular therapy is effective, so a measurement is taken before and after treatment for each individual and, once again, the question is asked: is the observed change a result of random chance, or is it real?

Attempts are made to answer such questions by the application of statistical procedures, although we should remember that statistics can never give absolute answers. We can, however, calculate the probability that an apparent change in a particular experimental measurement is the result of random variation, or chance, and if this probability is small, we can assume that the observed difference is real. We should, nevertheless, not forget that there is still a probability, although perhaps very small, that we may be wrong and that the observed difference *has* occurred by chance.

Statistics, as a subject, strikes fear into the hearts of many. In general, I believe, this is a fear of the unknown brought about by uncertainty. If approached slowly and methodically such fear can be overcome and a certain pleasure in handling data may be experienced. One of the major difficulties encountered by students seems to be deciding which of the many available statistical tests should be applied to a particular situation. Appendix V shows 'decision trees' for the various tests, offering a logical procedure for making an appropriate choice. I hope that these may be of some help in solving this problem.

Finally, I would like to express my thanks to friends and colleagues for encouragement and suggestions, particularly with regard to the examples and exercises which have been included in this book.

John McCall

1

Some Basic Statistical Principles

Contents
—The nature of descriptive and inferential statistics.
—Measures of central tendency: the mean and median.
—A measure of variability: the standard deviation.
—Populations and samples.
—Parameters and statistics.

Introduction

In general there are two basic reasons why statistics are necessary. Firstly, data may be collected simply to keep records or to convey information, and secondly, so that comparisons may be made, for example, between two different therapies in order to decide which is the more effective, or, perhaps, so that predictions may be made, i.e. inferences are drawn from the data. Thus two general categories may be recognized, which are referred to as *descriptive* and *inferential* statistics.[1]

Descriptive statistics

The methods of descriptive statistics are concerned with presenting data in a form which enables the general nature of the information

---

[1] Terms written in italics are defined or explained in the glossary in Appendix I.

to be assimilated more easily, for example, in the form of graphs, pie-charts, barcharts or histograms, which are various methods of display designed to give an instant visual impression. These techniques are described in Chapter 2. A few other simple statistics which also describe data and are, perhaps, a little more straight-forward are now described.

Percentages

It is, perhaps, worth a reminder at this stage of the way in which percentages are calculated. If we determine the frequency with which an event occurs, for example, if we measure the height of 50 young males and find that 15 of them are taller than 1.75 metres, and we wish to compare this with a second larger group of 80 in which we find that 28 are taller than 1.75 metres, we obviously cannot simply compare the frequency with which we find individuals taller than this value because the groups are different sizes. We can, however, compare the fraction in each case, that is $15/50 = 0.30$ and $28/80 = 0.35$. A more common approach is to quote the percentages, i.e. the frequencies are adjusted to the equivalent value if the sample had contained 100 individuals simply by multiplying the fraction by 100. Thus in the first case we have:

$$\frac{15}{50} \times 100 = 30\%$$

and in the second case:

$$\frac{28}{80} \times 100 = 35\%$$

The mean

In other circumstances we may have collected some data, for example, the resting heart rate, or, perhaps, the systolic blood pressure, of a large group of subjects in order to make an assessment of what is the 'norm'. When viewed as a page full of numbers it is very diffi-cult to gain a general impression of the nature of these measure-ments, so it is very useful if we can quote a 'characteristic' value. The most common approach is to calculate the average, which in the context of statistics is referred to as the *mean*.

The mean is calculated by obtaining the sum of all the measure-ments, i.e. by adding them all together, and dividing by the number of measurements.

Example 1.1

If we take six individuals, which we would refer to as a statis-tical *sample*, and measure the resting heart rate in each case, we may well find the following: 82, 76, 80, 71, 68 and 70. The mean is calculated by adding them all together and dividing by the number of measurements, in this case 6, i.e.

$$\bar{x} = \frac{82 + 76 + 80 + 71 + 68 + 70}{6}$$
$$= 74.5$$

The mean is sometimes referred to as a *measure of central tendency*.

The median

An alternative measure of central tendency is the *median*, which is simply the middle value. If the data are arranged in numerical order and we have an odd number of measurements, there is a unique mid-dle value, which is the median. If, however, we have an even number of observations, as in the example quoted above, there is no unique middle value, so, in that case, we take the average of the two middle values.

Example 1.2

$$68 \quad 70 \quad \underline{72 \quad 76} \quad 80 \quad 82$$

$$\text{Median} = \frac{72 + 76}{2} = 74$$

or, for an even number of values:

$$68 \quad 70 \quad 72 \quad \underline{76} \quad 80 \quad 82 \quad 83$$

$$\text{Median} = 76$$

If we have a large number of measurements and they are symmetrically distributed about the central value, then the mean and the median will be the same. In the example above, even though the sample is very small, they are close.

The mean is by far the most common measure of central tendency, but sometimes, if we have some extreme values the median is a better representation of the data. For example, imagine we are collecting for charity and 99 people give something between £1 and £2, with a mean of £1.50, and, let us assume, the median is also £1.50. If we then meet someone who has just won the national lottery and gives £1,000, the mean becomes £11.49, i.e.

$$\frac{(99 \times 1.50) + 1000}{100} = 11.49$$

whereas the median will be unchanged at £1.50, which is a much more 'characteristic' value for this set of data.

The median may, alternatively, be determined by a graphical method using a *cumulative frequency plot*, which is described in Chapter 2. This is perhaps the preferred approach if there is a large amount of data.

The mode

The mode, as the word suggests, is the most 'fashionable', or most common, value and although a modal value, or modal group in a

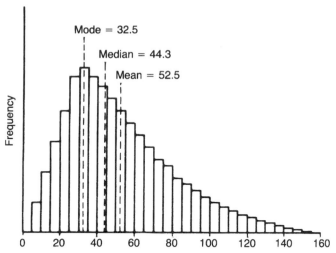

Figure 1.1 *An asymmetrical frequency distribution which is skewed to the right. If the distribution had been symmetrical, the mode, median and mean would have coincided*

histogram, can be identified, it is used principally with *nominal data* to indicate the category which occurs with the highest frequency. If a distribution is symmetrical the mean, median and mode will all coincide. In the case of a *skewed* distribution, that is one which is asymmetrical, or 'lop-sided', such as that shown in Figure 1.1, which is said to be 'skewed to the right', we can see that they do not coincide.

The standard deviation

In addition to the measure of central tendency, i.e. the mean (average) or median (middle value), it is very useful to have a measure of the way in which the data varies within the sample. Two sets of data may well have the same mean but one may be much more variable than the other, for example, consider the following measurements of systolic blood pressure. Set A and Set B represent repeated measurements by two different therapists on the same subject:

$$\text{(A)} \quad 121 \quad 120 \quad 118 \quad 122 \quad 119$$

$$\text{(B)} \quad 113 \quad 127 \quad 120 \quad 115 \quad 125$$

The mean of each group is 120 (you may care to confirm this with your calculator), yet one can see by simple inspection that Group A varies within a much narrower range (118 to 121) than Group B (113 to 127). Each group represents repeated measurements of the same quantity, i.e. the blood pressure of a particular individual. The first is said to be more precise than the second because it is less variable, or more reproducible. A measure of such variability is given by the *standard deviation*, which is discussed and defined in Chapter 4.

The standard deviation may be calculated, however, with your pocket calculator without worrying too much about its definition. Remember that the larger the value, the more variable, or less precise, are the measurements.

Try using your calculator to obtain the standard deviation of each of the above Sets A and B, known as *samples*. The standard deviation of a sample is given the symbol 's' by statisticians, and although it may well be obtained using the button marked 's' on the calculator, it is more likely that it will be marked σ_{n-1} or $x\sigma_{n-1}$. You should find that the values are 1.58 and 6.08 respectively. The subscript $(n-1)$ indicates that we are dealing with a *sample* rather than a *population*. The data represent samples because in each case we have six measurements only and, in principle, an infinite number of measurements could have been taken. Thus the population is infinite and the six measurements are a sample from that population. This point is discussed rather more fully later in this chapter in the section 'Inferential statistics' and in Chapter 4.

If it is feasible to measure the whole population, the standard deviation is given the symbol 'σ', and on the calculator the button marked σ, σ_n or $x\sigma_n$ would have been appropriate.

The coefficient of variation

Since the standard deviation is a measure of precision its size relative to the mean is clearly relevant, e.g. if the standard deviation is

2 and the mean is 500, the variability is very small relative to the mean and we have a precise set of measurements. If, however, the mean is only 5, the variability is large compared to the mean and we have a very imprecise set of measurements.

It is therefore often useful to quote the *coefficient of variation*, usually abbreviated to CV, rather than the standard deviation. This is simply the standard deviation represented as a percentage of the mean, e.g.

$$\text{Mean} = 25$$

$$\text{Standard deviation} = 2$$

$$\text{CV} = \frac{2}{25} \times 100$$

$$= 8\%$$

Thus the coefficient of variation in each case in the example considered in the previous section is 1.3% and 5.1% respectively, i.e.

$$\frac{1.58}{120} \times 100 = 1.3\% \quad \text{and} \quad \frac{6.08}{120} \times 100 = 5.1\%$$

Precision and accuracy

It is worth stressing at this point the distinction between *precision* and *accuracy*. To the lay person these terms are often considered to be synonymous, but they do have quite distinct meanings. Precision is a measure of reproducibility of measurements and accuracy is a measure of how close the measurement is to the true value. In general, of course, the latter is unknown and is the quantity that we are trying to determine with the help of statistics. Accuracy can, however, in certain circumstances, be tested by making a measurement of a quantity the value of which is already known, although this is not always possible.

It is perfectly possible to obtain a result which is very precise, but inaccurate. For example, if five people are given a goniometer and asked to measure the hip flexion of a particular patient, we would expect the five results to be very close to each other, i.e. a precise set of measurements. If, however, the goniometer had been wrongly calibrated, perhaps the angles starting at 10° rather than 0°, then all the measurements would be too large by 10°, so the mean would give us an inaccurate result. This would result in what is known as a *determinate error* or *gross error*, i.e. one which, in principle at least, may be detected, or 'determined', and hence eliminated.

The variation in the replicate measurements of hip flexion in the above example, ignoring the 10° error, is the result of random factors, which cannot be avoided, and for this reason are referred to as *indeterminate errors* or *random errors*. It is a measure of this variability which is given by the standard deviation.

Summary

DESCRIPTIVE STATISTICS. A name given to the methods by which data may be presented in a form which enables us to gain a general impression of its nature.

MEAN. The average or characteristic value of a set of data.

MEDIAN. The middle value.

MODE. The most common value.

STANDARD DEVIATION. A measure of variability.

ACCURACY. A measurement of how close a determination is to the true value.

PRECISION. A measure of reproducibility.

INDETERMINATE OR RANDOM ERROR. Variability of data which occurs as a result of random factors over which we have no control.

DETERMINATE OR GROSS ERRORS. Variability of data as a result of factors which, in principle, may be identified and eliminated.

Inferential statistics

If we wish to make predictions, or gather information about a very large group of individuals the size of which makes it impossible to measure individually, we would select, at random, a part of that group, which is referred to as a *sample*. The whole group is described as a *population*. The use of this term has its origin in history and currently refers to the total number of observations or measurements that are possible and is not restricted to people. Originally, many years ago, the needs of the population of a country, or state, or, perhaps, an army on the march, were estimated by considering the average needs of an individual, which were estimated from the needs of a small section of that population, i.e. a sample. The word 'statistics' seems to have its origin when referring to data collected by the state.

Thus, when it is not feasible to consider every member of the population, we would take our measurements, or observations, on a *sample*, selected at random from the population, and from these we would draw conclusions, or make inferences, about the population as a whole. Or, perhaps we might wish to compare two sets of data as suggested above. Such a procedure falls into the category of *inferential statistics*.

As an example, consider that we wish to know the average resting heart rate of the population of the United Kingdom. It is clearly impossible to measure the rate for every citizen in the country, so we would select a sample, which we would endeavour to choose at random. The average heart rate of our sample would then give us an estimate of the value for the population. It is reasonable to accept, although this can be demonstrated mathematically, that the larger the sample, the better will be the estimate of the mean for the population.

We should remember that the variation in the resting heart rates measured in different individuals is a biological variation and is not the result of random 'errors', such as would be seen if we measured the heart rate of a single individual several times. In general, the biological variation is much larger than any random error in measurement and the latter may usually be ignored when collecting data such as this with the purpose of showing the distribution within a population. The treatment may become a little involved if we consider both kinds of variation.

However, choosing a *random sample*, i.e. one in which every member of the population has an equal chance of being included, presents an additional problem. If we stand in the street and select, say, every fiftieth person to pass by and, assuming that we can induce them to rest for ten minutes, measure their heart rates, this may seem to be a reasonable approach. However, if we did this on a weekday, we may find that we have a preponderance of retired, or elderly, people because the younger members of the community are working at that time. Similarly, it would not be sensible to stand outside a junior school at finishing time because, once again, the age range of our sample would certainly not be representative of the population as a whole.

If the population is relatively small, for example, all the staff in a given hospital, we could assign a number to each and then use computer-generated random numbers to select the sample from that population. This procedure, however, is not feasible if the population is very large. It would clearly be impractical to assign numbers to all the citizens in the country in the way suggested above.

A lot has been written about the methods of obtaining random samples, but it is only possible, within the confines of this introductory text, to indicate very briefly some of the problems associated with their selection.

It is perhaps worth thinking a little at this stage about the concepts of a 'population' and a 'sample'. The same group of individuals can represent either a population, or a sample, depending upon the way in which a question is asked. For example, if we consider a class of 50 students in a university which has a total of 10,000 students. Two questions may be asked: (i) What are the average (mean) and standard deviation of the examination marks for this class? (ii) What are the average and standard deviation of the examination marks for all the students in the university?

The answer to the first question is easily obtained and, in this case, the 50 students in the class represent a population because the question is specific and applies to that group only. Unfortunately the terminology used by calculators is not consistent. The symbols σ and s are almost invariably used in printed texts for the standard deviation of the population and sample respectively, and although some calculators do use these symbols, others for some reason use σ_n and σ_{n-1}.

Thus the mean and standard deviation (using the button marked σ, σ_n or in some cases $x\sigma_n$) for all 50 students may be calculated. The class is small enough to be manageable, so we do not need to take a sample—although, of course, we could select, say, 10 students as a sample from that population, then the average mark for those 10 students would give us an estimate of the average for the whole class, and the standard deviation (s, σ_{n-1} or $x\sigma_{n-1}$) would give us an estimate of the value for all 50 students. In the circumstances, however, this would not only be unnecessary, but also not very sensible.

To answer the second question, the class of 50 students now becomes a sample, which we would have to assume is representative of the population of 10,000 students, and the mean ($\bar{x}$) and standard deviation (s) of that sample give us estimates of the mean (μ) and standard deviation (σ) of the population which comprises all 10,000 students in the university. The assumption that this is a random sample from the population would probably not be justified because students in a particular course may, in general, be more or perhaps less able than students on the whole. However, for the purpose of this example let us assume that it can be taken as a random sample. Thus we can do no better than make an estimate of the mean of the population, although the techniques of statistics enable us to assess how good this estimate might be. Such techniques are considered in Chapters 5 and 6.

Thus it can be seen that a given group of people, or measurements, may, depending on the way in which the question is asked, represent either a sample or a population.

We should note that a measurement or observation made on a sample is known as a *statistic* and will vary from one sample to another. For example, the mean mark for the class of 50 students considered above is an estimate of the population mean. If we chose another group of different students we would obtain another sample mean, which would also be an estimate of the population mean. We could continue and select several more groups and obtain several sample means, all of which we would expect to be close in value, but not identical. Each one of these is an independent estimate of the population mean.

The mean of the population, however, has a fixed value, because the population is fixed, although we do not know what it is, and it is referred to as a *parameter*.

To summarize, in general, sample *statistics* are estimates of population *parameters*.

It was mentioned above that a population comprises the total possible number of measurements or observations, which often, although it is not feasible to take them all, in principle, it is possible to do so. In some cases, however, where replicate measurements are taken on a single subject, e.g. measuring the angle of hip extension, the population is infinite because it is not possible to put a limit on the number of times that this measurement could be taken. If three repeated measurements were made, those three values would comprise the sample, whereas, in principle, the measurement could have been taken an infinite number of times, thus the population is infinite.

Summary

INFERENTIAL STATISTICS. Techniques by which we may (a) draw conclusions, or make inferences, about a population from data collected from a sample, or (b) compare two sets of data to determine whether they are significantly different from each other.

POPULATION. The total number of measurements or observations which it is theoretically possible to make. This may be finite (known or unknown) or infinite.

SAMPLE. A part of the population from which measurements or observations are made.

PARAMETER. The mean or standard deviation of a population. These have fixed values because the composition of the population is fixed. However, they are often unknown and are the very quantities that we are estimating from a sample.

STATISTIC. The mean or standard deviation of a sample. These do not have fixed values and will vary from one sample to another even though they are drawn from the same population. Each sample statistic is an independent estimate of the corresponding population parameter.

Exercises for Chapter 1

Exercise 1.1

Use your calculator for the following and quote the answers to one decimal place:

(a) In a particular university, a class contains 85 physiotherapy students in a particular year. The marks, as a percentage, for eight of these students, chosen at random, in their clinical placements were as follows:

55   65   60   45   50   50   70   80

Assume that the marks follow a normal distribution and estimate the mean, standard deviation and coefficient of variation of the class.

(b) Another, much smaller, class contains only ten students. The marks for this class are:

65   65   60   75   85   45   50   60   70   55

Determine the mean, standard deviation and coefficient of variation for this class.

Exercise 1.2

Determine the mean, standard deviation and coefficient of variation of each of the following sets of analytical measurements. Which is the more precise?

(a) 29.5   45.3   28.8   42.9   46.6   24.0   32.7   28.0
(b) 35.2   34.2   33.0   35.9   33.7   38.2   33.1   34.5

Exercise 1.3

(a) Calculate the mean, median and the standard deviation of the following sample:

26   32   21   24   25   24   28   26

(b) Change the last number from 26 to 66 and repeat the exercise. What do you notice?

Exercise 1.4

A goniometer was used to measure shoulder flexion in 37 patients suffering from 'frozen shoulder' and it was found 12 were less than 90° and 18 were less than 100°.

(a) What percentage of the patients exhibited a shoulder flexion (i) less than 90° and (ii) less than 100°?
(b) What percentage were between 90° and 100°?

Exercise 1.5

Determine (i) the mean and (ii) the median of the following data. Also (iii) determine the standard deviation and (iv) variance assuming they represent (a) a population and (b) a sample:

14   12   6   5   9   5   9   3   7   5   9   9   5   11   8   9   7

10   14   8

Exercise 1.6

A box contains four objects which weigh 25 g each, three objects of 15 g, and seven objects of 30 g. Calculate the mean weight and standard deviation.

2

Some Methods for Describing Data

Contents
—Piecharts, barcharts and histograms.
—Cumulative frequency plots.
—The median, quartiles, deciles and percentiles.
—Calculation of variance and standard deviation of a population and a sample.
—Degrees of freedom.

Introduction

Before considering the way in which data may be displayed, it will be useful to look at the different kinds of data which may be collected. Although often not important for descriptive purposes the distinction is, in general, important in the case of inferential statistics. Different types of data or scales of measurement may be summarized as follows.

Nominal data

Nominal data are sometimes referred to as 'categorical data' because information is categorized and it is not possible to quantify one category relative to another. To consider simple examples, 'male' and 'female' represent two categories, and individuals may be placed into one of them, or, perhaps, nationalities, British, French, Italian, etc. It is meaningless to refer to an average category.

Ordinal data

Ordinal data, as the name suggests, may be ranked in order. For example, if, in response to a particular question in a survey, people were asked to rank several institutions in order of their efficiency, it would not be feasible to say that one is 'twice (or perhaps three times) as good as another', but, simply, that one is better than another, because 'efficiency' cannot easily be quantified. So that putting the institutions into rank order, according to the opinion of the respondent, is all that can be accomplished. As another example, consider five candidates who have applied for a job are short-listed and interviewed. They could well be placed in rank order of suitability for the post, but, as above, it is not possible to say that one candidate is 'twice as good' as another.

Interval data

An interval scale is one in which the data are related by a uniform scale, e.g. the Celsius scale of temperature. The zero, however, is quite arbitrary and is set at the melting point of ice. Although a 5°C difference is the same between 5°C and 10°C as between 15°C and 20°C, we cannot say, for example, that 30°C is three times as warm as 10°C.

If, however, we were swimming in water, we may well describe it as very cold, cold, acceptable, warm or hot. The scale now becomes ordinal.

Ratio scale

Data measured on a scale with a true zero, such as weight or distance, are said to be on a 'ratio scale'. Measurements of length, for example, have a distinct zero, and we can safely say that 20 cm is twice as large as 10 cm.

In many cases, however, the distinction between interval data and ratio data is of no consequence.

Methods of displaying data

The general nature of a set of observations may be displayed using *piecharts*, *barcharts* or *histograms*. Piecharts and barcharts are simply two alternative methods of displaying the same information. They are used for *nominal* or *categorical data*, that is, individuals or events are counted and put into categories, thus the data is 'discrete', i.e. it is in the form of whole numbers.

The distinction between barcharts and histograms is sometimes a little confused. The latter, however, are used for *interval* data or *ratio data*, which is, in general, 'continuous', i.e. it includes measurements, and, unlike the 'discrete' data mentioned above, may be measured to as many significant figures (see Appendix II) as the measuring device will allow.

The lack of clear distinction between barcharts and histograms is, perhaps, because certain computer software, such as spreadsheets, will produce histograms only if the data are first put into groups or classes and the frequencies of occurrence in each class entered into the spreadsheet, whereupon, what is referred to as a 'barchart', but is actually a histogram, may be displayed.

Let us now look at some simple examples.

Piecharts

A piechart is used to display the way in which observations are divided into separate categories, i.e. for nominal data. For example, if a survey was conducted to determine the way in which the employees in a particular hospital travel to work, data such as that shown in the table below may be collected. The size of each 'slice' of the 'pie' is a measure of the size of that particular category as a fraction of the whole. This is illustrated in Figure 2.1. Since 25 from a total of 383 travel by bicycle, the size of the slice is 25/383 of the full

Method of travel	Number of employees
Bus	39
Train	185
Bicycle	25
Car	122
Motorcycle	12

Table 2.1

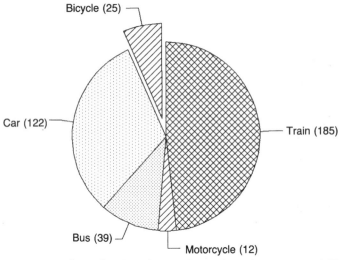

Figure 2.1 *A piechart showing the numbers of employees using different methods of travel to work. The data in this case are nominal, or categorical, and attention is drawn to the slice travelling by bicycle by 'exploding' it*

circle of 360°, i.e. the angle at the centre is drawn at (25/383) × 360° = 23.5°. Similarly, 122 travel by train, thus giving an angle of (122/383) × 360° = 114.7°, and so on. Note, also, that attention may be drawn to a particular segment by 'exploding' the piechart as shown.

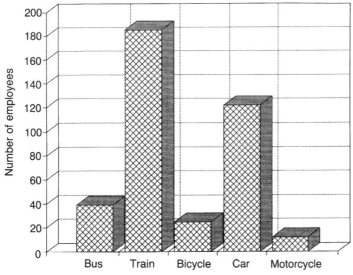

Figure 2.2 *A barchart showing the same information as Figure 2.1*

Barcharts

A barchart is simply an alternative method of presenting the same kind of data as a piechart. Figure 2.2 shows a barchart displaying the same data as the piechart considered above.

Summary

PIECHARTS AND BARCHARTS are alternative methods of displaying *nominal data* so that the relative sizes of each category may be clearly seen.

Remember that the order in which the categories are represented is arbitrary and that it is not possible to refer to a mean category.

Histograms with discrete data

A *histogram* may also be used to display 'discrete' data, i.e. whole numbers, where objects, events or people are counted. In this case,

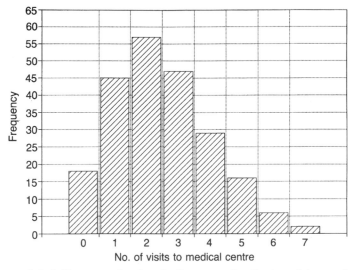

Figure 2.3 *A histogram showing the frequency distribution of the number of visits by employees to a medical centre. The data are on a ratio scale, but are discrete, i.e. can only be whole numbers because we are counting events*

however, the horizontal, or *x*-axis, is in the form of a scale, whereas in the case of the barchart, the order in which the categories are placed on this axis is totally arbitrary. An example may be seen in Figure 2.3 where the frequency of visits to the medical centre in a factory employing 220 people are displayed.

We can see from the first column in the histogram, representing zero visits, that this has occurred with a frequency of 18, i.e. 18 employees paid no visits to the medical centre. The second column shows that 45 employees paid one visit, 57 paid two visits, and so on.

Histograms with interval or ratio data

Both *interval* and *ratio* data may be displayed using a histogram. An example can be seen in Figure 2.4, which shows the distribution of measurements of the chest girth in a group of 250 male students. In this case each measurement has been placed into a 'class' or 'group'. The number of observations falling in each class is referred to as

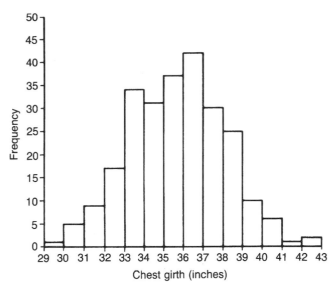

Figure 2.4 *A histogram showing the distribution of chest girth in 250 male students. The data are measured on a ratio scale and are continuous and have therefore been allocated to 'classes' or 'groups'*

the 'frequency', and the histogram represents a *frequency distribution*.

The data has been allocated to the 'classes' according to the value of each observation and the class boundaries, which are chosen arbitrarily, can be seen to be 29, 30, 31 . . . inches. Thus the classes are 29–30, 30–31, 31–32, etc. The simple convention, which is adopted by most computer statistical packages, such as MINITAB, is that any observation which lies on the boundary, e.g. 29.0 inches, is placed in the higher class, i.e. 29–30, which means, in reality, that all measurements equal to and greater than 29, but less than 30, are placed in this class, and so on for the other classes. For this reason the classes are sometimes represented as 29–<30, 30–<31, etc.

The classes, including the cumulative frequencies (the purpose of which will be explained later), are shown in Table 2.2. The first class includes one measurement lying between 29 and 'just below' 30, the second class includes five measurements between 30 and 'just below' 31, and so on.

Class	Frequency	Cumulative frequency	Percentage cumulative frequency
29–30	1	1	0.4
30–31	5	6	2.4
31–32	9	15	6.0
32–33	17	32	12.8
33–34	34	66	26.4
34–35	31	97	38.8
35–36	37	134	53.6
36–37	42	176	70.4
37–38	30	206	82.4
38–39	25	231	92.4
39–40	10	241	96.4
40–41	6	247	98.8
41–42	1	248	99.2
42–43	2	250	100.0

Table 2.2

Choice of class boundaries

The question which arises, of course, is how does one know what boundaries and how many classes to choose? The choice of boundaries is arbitrary and the most suitable number of classes depends on the quantity of data that has been collected. In the above example we have a large number of measurements so it is quite reasonable to have 14 classes, which is a relatively large number. If the number of measurements had been fairly small and a large number of classes were used, then it is likely that gaps would occur in the distribution, rather like missing teeth, where there are classes containing no observations. In general it is usually best to restrict the histogram to something like 8–12 classes, unless the number of observations is limited, in which case a smaller number would be more useful.

A cumulative frequency plot

The 'cumulative frequency' given in the table above represents the number of observations below the upper boundary of each

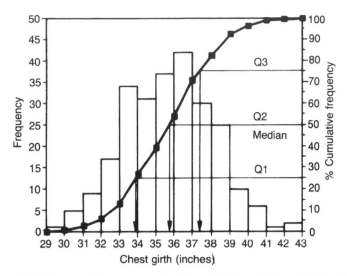

Figure 2.5 *The same histogram as that shown in Figure 2.4 to which has been added a cumulative frequency plot from which the first and third quartiles, Q1 and Q3 respectively, and the median may be determined*

particular class, i.e. 1, 1 + 5, 1 + 5 + 9, etc. This is often represented more conveniently as a percentage of the total, in this case of 250. When drawing the *cumulative frequency plot*, it is necessary, of course, to use a separate scale for the vertical axis on the plot, which is shown on the right-hand side, as can be seen in Figure 2.5. No observations are found to fall below 29, thus on the cumulative frequency plot the zero is placed at 29. Below 30 we find 0.4% of the observations, with 2.4% below 31, 6% below 32, and so on. The cumulative frequency plot can now be drawn, culminating with 100% at the upper class boundary of the highest class.

The median and the quartiles

It can be seen that each point on the cumulative frequency plot gives the percentage of the observations falling below a particular chest girth. Conversely, we can readily determine the measurement below which any given percentage of observations will be found. For example, the *median* is the 'middle' value, i.e. that value below which 50% of the observations are found.

The *quartiles*, represented by Q1, Q2 and Q3, give the values of the measurement, in this case the chest girth, below which a quarter, two quarters (i.e. one half) and three quarters of the observations are found. Thus, Q2 is the same as the median. We can see from Figure 2.5 that the median is about 35.8 inches, and the first and third quartiles, Q1 and Q3, are about 33.9 and 37.4 respectively. The range from Q1 to Q3 is referred to as the *interquartile range*, i.e. that range including the middle 50% of the observations.

Note that if the distribution is symmetrical, the median and the mean will be identical. In the above example, the distribution is approximately symmetrical, and it would be reasonable to accept that it would be so if a lot more data were to be collected.

Deciles and percentiles

Deciles and percentiles are alternatives to the quartiles when describing the distribution of data. They are determined in the same way as quartiles except deciles refer to tenths and percentiles refer to percentages rather than quarters. Thus the second decile, for example, is that value below which two tenths of the observations are found, and the fifth decile is the same as the second quartile and the median, that is the value below which five tenths, two quarters or one half of the observations are found. Similarly the sixtieth percentile, for example, is the value below which 60% of the observations are found. Clearly the fiftieth percentile, as with the fifth decile, is the same as the median.

Measures of dispersion

The standard deviation and the variance

As mentioned in Chapter 1, the *standard deviation* is a measure of the way in which a group of measurements, or other data, vary as a result of random factors, i.e. it is a measure of 'dispersion' or 'spread'. Remember that the more variable the data, the larger the value of the standard deviation.

The *variance*, however, which is the square of the standard deviation, is the more fundamental measure from a mathematical point of view although it is not often quoted. For a population the *variance* is defined as follows:

$$\sigma^2 = \frac{1}{N} \sum (x - \mu)^2 \tag{2.1}$$

where μ is the mean and x is the *random variable*, that is the observed, or measured quantity, N is the number of observations and $\sum$ (a capital sigma) means 'the sum of'. Sigma (lower case) squared (σ^2) is used to signify the variance. Note that the variance is the average sum of the squares of the differences between each observation and the mean. The reason that the square is taken is that the simple sum of the differences, i.e.

$$\sum (x - \mu) \tag{2.2}$$

must be zero, because of the way in which the mean is calculated, i.e. the sum of the positive differences must be equal to the negative differences. If, however, the square is taken, this is not the case, because the square of a negative number is positive.

A word of warning: the sum of the squares of the differences between each observation and the mean is often simply referred to as the 'sum of the squares'.

The standard deviation

The standard deviation, i.e. the square root of the variance, is, in general, a much more useful measure of dispersion or variability and is thus defined as:

$$\sigma = \sqrt{\frac{1}{N} \sum (x - \mu)^2} \tag{2.3}$$

The reason that this is more convenient is because it has the same dimensions as the mean, e.g. if we collect data comprising, say, weights of people, the dimensions, or units, of x (the weights of individuals), together with the mean and the standard deviation will all be the same, namely, kg. The units of the variance, however, will be kg^2.

The standard deviation calculated from a sample

The above definition refers to the calculation of the standard deviation of a *population*, i.e. where we have access to and can measure every member of that population, and μ is the mean. If it is necessary, as is usually the case, to estimate the standard deviation of the population from a value calculated from a sample, that is, a part of the population, then a slightly different definition is employed, namely:

$$s = \sqrt{\frac{1}{(n-1)} \sum (x - \bar{x})^2} \qquad (2.4)$$

Note the differences. The population *parameter*, σ, has been replaced by s, a sample *statistic*, which is an estimate of σ calculated from the sample, and μ has been replaced by $\bar{x}$, the sample mean. Also, N has been replaced by $(n-1)$, the number of *degrees of freedom*, where n is the size of the sample. The number of 'degrees of freedom' represents the number of the variables which may be altered independently whilst maintaining the total sum. For example, consider the following sample: 5, 3, 4, 6. The total (sum) is 18. Thus, if any three of the values are fixed, e.g. 5, 3 and 4, then, if the total is to remain at 18, the fourth value can only be 6.

It can be shown mathematically that a better estimate of σ is obtained if the number of degrees of freedom, rather than the number of observations, is employed in the calculation. This gives a slightly larger value than by dividing by n, the number of observations making up the sample. The increased variability arises from the fact that μ (the population mean) is not known and is estimated by the mean of the sample $(\bar{x})$.

Clearly, for large samples, the difference between dividing by n and dividing by $(n-1)$ becomes negligible and, as a general rule of thumb, if the sample size is greater than about the 30 the sample standard deviation may be taken to be the population value.

Calculation of means and standard deviations

Remember that the above are definitions of the standard deviations of a population and a sample and are quoted simply to show the nature of these quantities. It is exceedingly tedious to calculate them directly from the definitions, although it is, of course, possible, but unnecessary, because relatively simple modern calculators will enable you to compute them much more easily. By the way, it is well worth taking a little time to become familiar with your calculator so that you are able to make full use of it.

Thus the standard deviation of a sample (using the button s, σ_{n-1} or $x\sigma_{n-1}$) or a population (σ, σ_n or $x\sigma_n$) may readily be computed. Remember that calculators generate the standard deviation so that in the event that the variance is required, this must be squared.

Should it be the case that only a very basic calculator is at hand, the definition of the standard deviation may be modified into a rather different form which makes the calculation a little more simple, namely:

$$\sigma = \sqrt{\frac{1}{N}\left(\sum x^2 - N\mu^2\right)} \qquad \text{for a population}$$

$$\text{or} \quad s = \sqrt{\frac{1}{(n-1)}\left(\sum x^2 - n\bar{x}^2\right)} \quad \text{for a sample}$$

(2.5)

Remember that if it is feasible to calculate the mean of the whole population, this is done in exactly the same way as for a sample, but it is given the symbol μ rather than $\bar{x}$.

Calculation of the mean and standard deviation from grouped data

Let us assume that we wish to calculate the mean and standard deviation for the data referring to the chest girth of 250 students which was considered earlier in the chapter. These data are shown in Table 2.2 and, in the form of a histogram, in Figure 2.4. Since the 'raw data' are not available it is not possible to calculate the exact mean and the only course of action that is open to us is to assume that all the observations in a given class have the value of the mid-point of the class, which is referred to as the *class mark*, e.g.

$$\text{Mean} = \frac{\sum xf}{n}$$

$$= \frac{(29.5 \times 1) + (30.5 \times 5) + (31.5 \times 9) + \cdots}{250}$$
$$+ (41.5 \times 1) + (42.5 \times 2)$$

$$= 35.7 \text{ in}$$

where x is the class mark, f the frequency in each class, i.e. the number of measurements which fall within the range of that particular class, and n the total number of measurements.

It can be seen that the calculated mean (35.7) is very close to the value estimated for the median (35.8) from the cumulative frequency plot in Figure 2.5. This suggests that the distribution of frequencies is symmetrical.

Many hand calculators will enable you to perform the above calculation directly, together with that for the standard deviation. The procedure is as follows: Select the SD mode on the calculator and ensure that the memories used for the statistical calculations are empty—this is usually achieved by pressing the SHIFT button followed by AC (all clear). Type in the first class mark (the mid-point of the class), the multiply button, the frequency and then the normal data entry button that is used for statistical calculations. Follow this by the second class mark, multiply button, the frequency of the second class and the data entry button, and so on until all the classes and frequencies have been entered. For example:

$$29.5 \times 1 \quad \text{data entry}$$
$$30.5 \times 5 \quad \text{data entry, etc.}$$

Thus 29.5 is entered into the calculator once, 30.5 is entered five times, and so on. The same result may, of course, be obtained, although rather more laboriously, by simply entering 29.5 once and then 30.5 five times, until all the class marks have been entered the appropriate number of times.

The mean and standard deviation may now be obtained in the usual manner by pressing the appropriate buttons. Strictly, the 250 students represent a sample, but because this sample is so large, the difference between the standard deviation obtained by treating it as a population and by treating it as a sample is very small. You should find these to be 2.405 and 2.410, respectively. If corrected to 2 decimal places they become the same, namely, 2.41.

Symbols

It is perhaps convenient at this point to summarize some of the symbols that are commonly encountered.

$$\sum x = x_1 + x_2 + x_3 + \cdots$$

$$\sum x_1^2 = x_1^2 + x_2^2 + x_3^2 + \cdots$$

$$\left(\sum x\right)^2 = (x_1 + x_2 + x_3 + \cdots)^2$$

$$\sum (x - \bar{x})^2 = (x_1 - \bar{x})^2 + (x_2 - \bar{x})^2 + (x_3 - \bar{x})^2 + \cdots$$

$$\sum xy = x_1 y_1 + x_2 y_2 + x_3 y_3 + \cdots$$

$\bar{x}$ = the mean of a sample,

μ = the mean of a population,

s = the standard deviation of a sample,

s^2 = the variance of a sample,

σ = the standard deviation of a population,

σ^2 = the variance of a population.

Parameters and statistics

Remember that population parameters are generally represented by Greek letters and sample statistics by Roman letters, and that the latter are estimates of the former.

Summary

PIECHARTS AND BARCHARTS are alternative ways of displaying category or *nominal data*. *Continuous data* may be displayed in the form of a histogram, which is similar in appearance to a barchart.

HISTOGRAMS may be constructed from *discrete data*, e.g. when counting individuals, or events, such as visits to a medical centre, and thus must be represented by whole numbers, or from *continuous data*, e.g. measurements, such as chest girth of a group of subjects. They are prepared by grouping the data into a number of 'classes' and displaying the frequency with which observations are made within the limits of each class.

THE MEDIAN is the middle value of a set of data, i.e. that value below which 50% of the observations or measurements occur. Like the mean, it gives a value which is characteristic of the data, but is rather more representative than the mean if the data contains some extreme values.

A CUMULATIVE FREQUENCY PLOT, sometimes referred to as an 'ogive', offers a convenient method of determining the median and the quartiles.

THE VARIANCE is a measure of the dispersion or spread of the data.

THE STANDARD DEVIATION is the square root of the variance—a rather more convenient measure of the dispersion or spread of the data.

Exercises for Chapter 2

Exercise 2.1

The time (days) required for 20 patients to recover from a particular injury was recorded as follows:

17   19   16   21   20   18   10   14   28   15

11   12   14   32   15   36   24   13   27   22

(a) Determine the mean, standard deviation and variance.
(b) Construct a histogram to display these data with the first class mark (class mid-point) at 10 and a class width of 4.
(c) From the appearance of the histogram would you conclude that these data follow a normal distribution?
(d) Draw a cumulative frequency plot and hence determine the median.
(e) What percentage of patients would you expect to recover within three weeks?

Exercise 2.2

Systolic blood pressure measurements were taken from ten patients selected at random from those attending a hospital clinic. The following results were obtained (mmHg):

  119   131   138   134   133   127   125   116   119   134

(a) How many degrees of freedom are there in this sample?
(b) Estimate the average systolic blood pressure of the patients in the clinic. Also, estimate the variance and the standard deviation.

Exercise 2.3

The systolic blood pressure of a sample of 25 young adult males was measured and found to be as follows (mmHg):

  127   117   126   123   123   125   115   118   120

  119   112   108   131   115   121   118   121   122

  125   113   123   118   127   122   120

(a) Display these data in the form of a histogram with the first class mark (class mid-point) at 108 and a class width of 4.
(b) Draw a cumulative frequency plot and use it to obtain values for the median and the interquartile range.
(c) Use the cumulative frequency plot to estimate a 'reference range', i.e. the range within which 95% of the young adult male

population would be expected to be included. Do you think that this would yield a reliable estimate of the reference range?

Exercise 2.4

The resting heart rate of 64 apparently healthy young women was measured in beats per minute (bpm) with the following results:

Class boundaries	Frequency
54–58	1
58–62	4
62–66	7
66–70	12
70–74	14
74–78	12
78–82	6
82–86	5
86–90	2
90–94	1

Plot a cumulative frequency curve and hence estimate the resting heart rate above which 10% of the population would be expected to be found.

Estimate also the mean and standard deviation.

Exercise 2.5

The following data represent the skinfold thicknesses of 20 male subjects measured (mm) at the triceps mid-point:

7.5   13.7   8.7   10.1   9.2   10.4   10.7   10.0   11.7   10.3

11.2   12.9   11.4   11.8   9.8   6.7   9.2   9.6   12.1   7.1

(a) Determine the mean and standard deviation of the sample.
(b) Construct a histogram to display these data.
(c) Draw a cumulative frequency plot and hence determine (i) the median (ii) the interquartile range (iii) the third decile and (iv) the sixtieth percentile.
(d) Estimate the skinfold thickness above which it would be expected to find 10% of the population.

3

The Linear Relationship between Data Collected in Pairs. Correlation, Regression and Prediction

Contents
—Correlation and the Pearson product moment correlation coefficient.
—The Spearman correlation coefficient for ranked data.
—Kendall's coefficient of concordance to compare more than two sets of ranked scores.
—The regression equation and the 'line of best fit'.

Introduction

When data are collected in pairs, the relationship between the observations or measurements, or as they are often called, the 'variables', is usually of interest. The general nature of such a relationship may often be gained by producing a 'scatterplot' i.e. labelling the two sets of data x and y respectively and simply plotting the points against the two scales on a graph. Conventionally the horizontal axis (the 'abscissa') is labelled x, and the vertical axis (the 'ordinate') is labelled y.

In some cases one of the variables is under the control of the observer, or is fixed in some way or another, and is referred to as the *independent variable*, whilst the second variable, which depends upon it, is called the *dependent variable*. For example, if the weight of infants was measured and related to age, the latter is clearly the independent variable since weight is obviously dependent on age rather than vice versa. Similarly, if we consider life expectancy and the number of cigarettes smoked per day, once again, the latter is clearly the independent variable. Also by convention, when plotting a graph, the independent variable is placed on the x (horizontal) axis.

In other cases, the choice of x and y is totally arbitrary, i.e. one does not depend upon the other. For example, if the examination score for a group of students for, say, physiology and anatomy were to be correlated, neither mark could be considered to be an independent variable with the other depending upon it. In this case the allocation of x and y would be arbitrary and it would not matter which was plotted on which axis.

The correlation coefficient

The *correlation coefficient*, or to give it its full title, the 'Pearson product moment correlation coefficient', is a measure of the linear relationship between two variables such as those mentioned above. It is given the symbol r and is defined in such a way that it may only take values between -1.00 and $+1.00$. If $r = +1.00$, this indicates that there is perfect positive correlation, i.e. as x increases, y increases in an exact linear relationship with the points in the scatter diagram lying exactly on a straight line. If $r = -1.00$, there is perfect negative correlation, i.e. the points also lie exactly on a straight line but y decreases as x increases.

The definition of the correlation coefficient

The correlation coefficient is defined as follows:

$$r = \frac{1}{n-1} \sum \frac{(x - \bar{x})(y - \bar{y})}{s_x s_y} \tag{3.1}$$

If you are interested in the reason for the definition being in this form, an explanation is given in Appendix IV.

Examples of various correlation coefficient values

Figures 3.1 and 3.2 represent data with a correlation coefficient of +1.0 and −1.0 respectively. In Figure 3.3, the value is 0.81. Although there is considerable scatter about the line, it can be seen that a general trend exists, i.e. as x increases, y also increases.

In Figure 3.4, however, the points in the scatter plot appear to be at random, i.e. no relationship exists between the two sets of data. The correlation coefficient is very close to zero.

Figure 3.5 shows an example in which the value of the correlation coefficient is zero although a very well-defined relationship clearly exists between the two variables. The point here is that the relationship is not linear. This is, of course, an extreme example and is unlikely to be met in practice.

We should remember at this stage that correlation does not imply causation. It is perfectly possible that both variables may change in a similar fashion for completely independent reasons. There are many examples to illustrate this, one of the most famous being the strong correlation that was found to exist between the number of

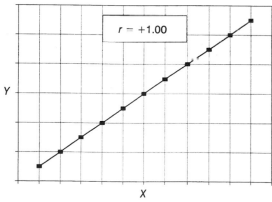

Figure 3.1 *An example of perfect positive correlation*

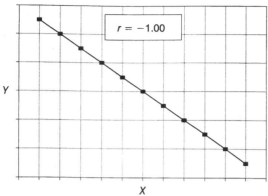

Figure 3.2 *An example of perfect negative correlation*

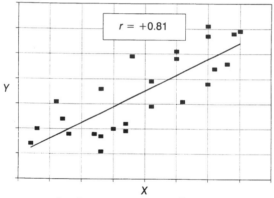

Figure 3.3 *An example of strong positive correlative*

divorces in this country and the number of apples imported. Nobody would believe that importing apples causes divorce.

Calculation of the correlation coefficient

Many hand calculators will do this very simply when in the 'linear regression mode', usually designated MODE LR, and, of course, there are many computer packages which may be used.

Alternatively, if only a basic calculator is at hand, it can readily be shown that the definition of r (Equation 3.1) may be rearranged into

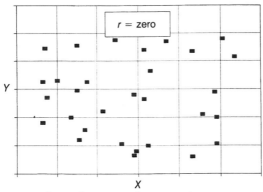

Figure 3.4 *No relationship exists between the two variables and, as a consequence, the correlation coefficient is zero*

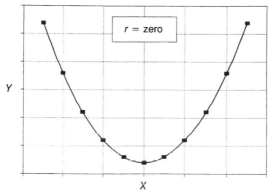

Figure 3.5 *An example of data where the correlation coefficient is zero even though a strong relationship exists between the two variables. The point is that the relationship is not linear*

the following form, which enables the computation to be performed a little more easily:

$$r = \frac{1}{n-1} \frac{\sum xy - n\bar{x}\bar{y}}{s_x s_y} \qquad (3.2)$$

where:
$\bar{x}$ and $\bar{y}$ are the means of x and y,
s_x and s_y are the standard deviations of x and y,
n is the number of pairs of observations,
$\sum xy = x_1 y_1 + x_2 y_2 + x_3 y_3 + \cdots x_n y_n$.

The value obtained is a measure of *linear* correlation. The square of this coefficient, r^2, which is referred to as the coefficient of determination, is a measure of the fraction of the relationship which may be explained by a linear equation. It is thus clear that the interpretation of the correlation coefficient must be undertaken with a little caution and should not be used to justify an assumption of a truly linear relationship. If the points clearly lie on a gentle curve, a value for r close to unity may be obtained.

When calculating the correlation coefficient it is not important which variable is considered to be x and which is y. It will be seen later, however, when considering linear regression, which is the procedure by which the best straight line is drawn through the points on a graph, that often it *is* important to make the distinction.

Consider the following example, where the data give the height and weight of ten individuals. We would expect, of course, that the two would be related and that taller people would tend to weigh more than shorter people. The correlation coefficient confirms that this is so.

Example 3.1

Height/m: 1.68 1.69 1.70 1.82 1.75 1.80 1.81 1.90 1.91 1.92

Weight/kg: 66.9 70.0 67.7 67.9 68.1 72.0 71.2 71.0 74.5 76.3

If we arbitrarily let the height be represented by x and the weight by y, the following may be obtained:

$$\bar{x} = 1.798 \qquad \bar{y} = 70.56$$

$$\sum xy = 1,270.70 \qquad n = 10$$

$$s_x = 0.0919 \qquad s_y = 3.094$$

so that, using Equation 3.2, we may now calculate the correlation coefficient:

$$r = \frac{1}{(10-1)} \left(\frac{1,270.70 - 10(1.798)(70.56)}{(0.0919)(3.094)} \right) = 0.793$$

This indicates that there is, as expected, a strong correlation between height and weight.

Having calculated the correlation coefficient and found it to be 0.793, it is necessary to consider the significance of this value. In other words, we ask the question: does this value for r represent a real correlation or could it have occurred by chance? We know that the closer the value is to unity, the stronger is the relationship, but we need to consider the calculated value a little more closely.

The significance of the correlation

Following any statistical test where an inference is made, it is said that the *significance* of the result is determined. In simple terms, referring to the correlation coefficient, r, remembering that, because of the way that it is defined, it may only take values between ± 1.0, we ask the question: is the observed value too large for us to accept that it has occurred by chance when there really is no correlation and the actual value is zero?

The approach to this problem is to quote two hypotheses. The null hypothesis, given the symbol H_0, which asserts that the population value for the correlation coefficient (ρ) is really zero and that the value we have observed (r) has occurred by chance, and the alternative, often called the experimental, hypothesis, H_1, which asserts that the value is not zero. Note the usual convention that Greek letters are used to represent the population *parameters* and Roman letters to represent sample *statistics*.

The hypotheses are usually written as follows:

$$H_0: \quad \rho = 0$$

$$H_1: \quad \rho \neq 0$$

Remember that the population is the total number of observations which, in principle, it would be possible to make. In Example 3.1, this would be the measurements of the heights and weights of all the citizens in the country, or perhaps in the world, which is clearly not feasible.

Thus, we hypothesize that the population correlation coefficient (ρ) is zero, and determine, from the appropriate tables (Table G in Appendix VI) the probability that a value as far from zero as 0.793 would occur entirely by chance when n, the number of pairs of observations or measurements, is 10. If this probability is low, we accept that it is unlikely that it has occurred by chance and that a real correlation does exist. If this probability is high, we accept that, indeed, it has happened by chance and that the observed value of the correlation coefficient is the result of random variation over which we have no control, and therefore there is not a real correlation between the two variables.

The next question is, of course: what do we mean by low and high? The usual cut-off point is taken to be 5%, or a probability of 0.05, so that, if the probability of the observed value occurring by chance, when the null hypothesis is true, is below 5%, we accept that the result is not a chance happening and that a real correlation exists. This is called the *level of significance* and is often represented as $\alpha = 0.05$.

Table G gives the critical values of the correlation coefficient for various sample sizes. We should note that the number of degrees of freedom is $(n - 2)$—this is because, when considering a point in a scatter plot, two coordinates are necessary to define its position.

From the table, for a two-way test with a sample of 10, the *critical values* of r are given:

r	P
0.549	0.10
0.632	0.05
0.716	0.02
0.765	0.01
0.847	0.002

This means that *if* no correlation exists, i.e. $\rho =$ zero, then in a sample of size 10, r may take a value as large as 0.549 with a probability of 0.10, or 10%, and as large as 0.632 with a probability of 0.05, or 5%, and so on. Thus the larger is the value of r, the smaller is the probability that it has occurred by chance and the greater is the probability that it represents a real correlation.

The value obtained in Example 3.1, namely 0.793, lies between the critical values at $P = 0.01$ (0.765) and $P = 0.002$ (0.847), so that we would report that there is a probability of between 0.2% and 1% that this value has arisen by chance. Since this probability is low—well below the chosen significance level of 5%—we have sufficient evidence to reject the null hypothesis in favour of the alternative and accept that a true correlation exists.

It is better to quote a 'P value' rather than simply to report that the correlation is significant at 5% because in the latter case, no distinction is made between a probability of, say, 0.045, which is only a little below 5%, and 0.001, which is very much below 5%. Thus, more information is provided and a reader will gain a better idea of the strength of the correlation.

In Example 3.1, therefore, the result would be written:

$$0.002 < P < 0.01$$

It is worth noting that, if working at the 5% level of significance, we are saying that we are prepared to accept a 5% chance of being wrong if we reject the null hypothesis and conclude that a real correlation exists. This is, of course, because there is a 5% probability that the observed value has, in fact, occurred by chance and there really is no correlation.

One- and two-way tests

In Example 3.1 we performed what is variously known as a 'two-way', 'two-tailed' or 'non-directional test', that is to say we were making no assumption regarding the sign of the correlation coefficient. Our conclusion was that there is a probability of between 0.2% and 1% that the value of r would differ from zero by 0.793, or more, if the null hypothesis is true, i.e. $\rho = $ zero. That is, it is greater than +0.793 or less than −0.793.

It would, however, be reasonable for us to expect that weight and height would increase together, i.e. the correlation would be positive, so we do not really need to concern ourselves with the possibility of it having a value of −0.793. We can, therefore, perform a 'one-way', 'one-tailed' or 'directional test', where we test only the probability that r might be as large as +0.793 by chance. The hypotheses would then be written:

$$H_0: \ \rho = 0$$
$$H_1: \ \rho > 0$$

and we take the critical values given in Table G for a one-way test where the significance level for a given value of r is halved.

The general arguments used above when considering the significance of the correlation coefficient are the same for all statistical tests of significance and will crop up again in later chapters.

Correlation of non-parametric data

If we have collected some data and have reason to believe that it differs considerably from the *normal distribution*, or, perhaps, it is *ordinal* in nature, i.e. the observations are in rank order only, a non-parametric correlation coefficient should be used. In this circumstance it is the ranks which are correlated rather than the raw data.

The Spearman correlation coefficient for ranked data

The most convenient method of calculating the Spearman coefficient is to rank each set of data separately and determine the normal (Pearson) correlation coefficient between the *ranks* with a calculator. However, the following formula is often quoted for the calculation because it was considered to be rather easier to use in the days before calculators were commonly at hand, and for that reason is mentioned here:

$$r_s = 1 - \frac{6 \sum d^2}{(n^3 - n)} \tag{3.3}$$

where:

r_s = the Spearman rank order correlation coefficient,
d = the difference between the rank of each pair of observations,
$\sum d^2$ = the sum of the squares of these differences,
n = the number of pairs of observations.

The rationale for this equation is as follows: Spearman noted that for any set of rankings, the sum of the ranks, that is the sum of the first n integers, is $n(n + 1)/2$, for example, for the ranks 1 to 5 the sum is given by:

$$1 + 2 + 3 + 4 + 5 = \frac{5(5 + 1)}{2} = 15$$

Also the sum of the squares of the ranks, or the squares of the first n integers is $n(n + 1)(2n + 1)/6$:

$$1^2 + 2^2 + 3^2 + 4^2 + 5^2 = \frac{5(5 + 1)(10 + 1)}{6} = 55$$

Thus, because the data are ranked, $\sum x$ and $\sum y$ were replaced in the Pearson formula by $n(n + 1)/2$ and $\sum x^2$ and $\sum y^2$ by $n(n + 1)(2n + 1)/6$. But, it should be stressed that, strictly, this is only the case if there are no tied ranks (see the following example for the method of treating tied ranks). Although a rather elaborate procedure was developed to correct for tied ranks, there seems to be little point in calculating the Spearman coefficient using the above equation and making the correction when it can be calculated in a much more straightforward manner using the Pearson formula using the ranks, rather than the raw data.

If there are only few tied ranks there is little difference between r_s, calculated as above, and the value obtained by correlating the ranks with the Pearson formula. However, with a large number of tied ranks, the difference can be rather more important. Consider the following example where we shall calculate the Spearman coefficient using the above formula and also use the Pearson formula on the ranks.

Example 3.2

Imagine that there are two tests which use slightly differing criteria for assessment of speech in children and we wish to compare them. Six children are assessed using a five-point scale by each test with the following results:

Child	Test X	Test Y
A	5	4
B	3	2
C	5	4
D	4	3
E	3	3
F	3	2

Consider the results from Test X. If these are ranked in order we can see that the three lowest values of 3 share the ranks 1, 2 and 3 and each is therefore allocated an average rank, namely, 2. The value 4 takes the rank 4, and the two values of 5 share the ranks 5 and 6 and each is therefore ranked at 5.5.

Child:	B	E	F	D	A	C
Test score (X):	3	3	3	4	5	5
Rank:		1 & 2 & 3		4		5 & 6
Average rank:	2	2	2	4	5.5	5.5

Similarly for Test Y so that the ranks may be listed for each child:

Child	Test Rank X	Rank Y	Difference d	d^2
A	5.5	5.5	0	0
B	2	1.5	0.5	0.25
C	5.5	5.5	0	0
D	4	3.5	0.5	0.25
E	2	3.5	−1.5	2.25
F	2	1.5	0.5	0.25

$$\sum d^2 = 3$$
$$n = 6$$

Substituting $\sum d^2 = 3$ and $n = 6$ in Equation 3.3 we find:

$$r_s = 1 - \frac{6 \times 3}{(6^3 - 6)} = 0.914$$

If, however, we simply correlate the *ranks* X, Y using the normal Pearson equation (Equation 3.2) or a calculator in the linear regression we find that:

$$r_s = 0.904$$

This example was chosen to indicate the method of dealing with shared ranks and also, although the difference is not very large, to illustrate that, strictly, Equation 3.3 does not give the correct result because of the tied ranks.

The significance of r_s

The interpretation of r_s is not quite so straightforward as in the case of Pearson's r because ranked data cannot be normally distributed, although there is the advantage that we no longer make the assumption that the underlying relationship between the two variables is linear. A set of critical values for r_s is given in Table H in Appendix VI. Similar tables appear in various texts although it will be found that some of them do vary slightly from one to another. However, once the sample size is greater than about 12, the values quoted in tables for r_s and r are very close to each other.

If we refer to Table H we see that the value obtained in Example 3.2 ($r_s = 0.904$) is larger than the critical value given at the 5% level of significance when $n = 6$ for a one-way test.

Referring to Example 3.2, we would be looking for a positive correlation so a one-way test is appropriate, i.e.

$$H_0: \ \rho = 0$$

$$H_1: \ \rho > 0$$

and reference to Table H shows that the critical value for $n = 6$ at the 5% level of significance is 0.829. Either value obtained in this example is above this critical value, although strictly we should use the one obtained with the Pearson formula ($r_s = 0.904$) because of the tied ranks. We would therefore conclude that there is a significant correlation between the results of Test X and Test Y. In other words, there is a less than 5% probability that the apparent correlation has occurred by chance.

Be careful not to become confused by the fact that the rank correlation coefficient may be calculated using the Pearson formula— it is still calculated on the *ranks* and therefore the significance should be assessed with reference to Table H for the Spearman coefficient.

Warning

We should remember that a correlation coefficient of $+1.0$ for either r_s or r simply means that the correlation is perfect, i.e. as one variable increases, the other also increases in exact proportion. It *does not* mean that the two sets of scores are equivalent. Consider the following example, which is extreme but has been included to make the point:

Example 3.3

Two assessors rated five subjects on a ten-point scale with the following scores:

$$\text{Assessor 1:} \quad 10 \quad 9 \quad 8 \quad 7 \quad 6$$
$$\text{Assessor 2:} \quad \ 5 \quad 4 \quad 3 \quad 2 \quad 1$$

The correlation coefficient (either r_s or r) will be found to be $+1.0$, indicating perfect correlation, yet no one would conclude that the two assessments are equivalent.

Note

Be careful not to become confused if data are represented in different ways, e.g. for the subjects in Example 3.2 the scores for each test are shown as rows and in Example 3.3 the scores for each test (assessor) are shown as columns.

Let us now look at another example to illustrate that, although in certain circumstances it is sensible to calculate a ranked correlation coefficient, some information about the raw data is lost:

Example 3.4

Consider a pair of scores for five subjects similar to those in Example 3.3:

$$\text{Assessor 1:} \quad 2 \quad 3 \quad 4 \quad 9 \quad 10$$
$$\text{Assessor 2:} \quad 2 \quad 3 \quad 4 \quad 5 \quad 10$$

The Spearman rank correlation coefficient $r_s = +1.0$, because, of course, the fourth scores of 9 and 5 respectively both have the rank 4, so that the ranks for each subject are identical in each set of scores. The Pearson correlation coefficient, r, does not consider the scores 9 and 5 to be equivalent and a value of 0.872 is obtained.

Note: If we use the Pearson formula on the *ranks* we also get a value of $r_s = +1.0$.

In the above examples, we have calculated r_s from ranks allocated to ratings on a scale that cannot be considered to be an interval or ratio, perhaps in the form 1 = very poor, 2 = poor, 3 = medium, 4 = good and 5 = very good. It may equally well be calculated when subjects are simply put into rank order as in Exercise 3.1 at the end of this chapter.

Non-parametric comparison of more than two samples— the Kendall coefficient of concordance

Both the Pearson and the Spearman correlation coefficients only investigate the association between two groups or samples. A circumstance may well arise where we require to see whether significant agreement occurs in ranking by more than two assessors. The *Kendall coefficient of concordance* permits such a comparison.

Consider a situation where four therapists assess the same five children and rank them in order of speech ability. We wish to determine whether there is general agreement between them. Once again, the procedure is best explained with an example:

Example 3.5

The five subjects were ranked by the four therapists as follows:

			Child		
	A	B	C	D	E
Therapist W	1	2	3	4	5
X	1	2	3	4	5
Y	2	4	3	1	5
Z	1	2	5	3	4
Rank totals	5	10	14	12	19

Firstly the mean rank total for each subject is calculated:

$$\text{Mean rank total} = M_T = \frac{5 + 10 + 14 + 12 + 19}{5} = 12$$

The sum of the squares of the differences between each rank total (R_T) and the mean rank total (M_T) is given the symbol S and is a measure of the variability of those totals:

$$
\begin{aligned}
S &= \sum (\text{Rank total} - \text{Mean rank total})^2 \\
&= \sum (R_T - M_T)^2 \\
&= (5 - 12)^2 + (10 - 12)^2 + (14 - 12)^2 + (12 - 12)^2 \\
&\quad + (19 - 12)^2 \\
&= 49 + 4 + 4 + 0 + 49 \\
&= 106
\end{aligned}
$$

This is compared with the maximum possible value for the sum of the squares (S_{max}) which it can be shown is given by:

$$S_{max} = \tfrac{1}{12} k^2 (n^3 - n)$$

where:
$k = 4 =$ the number of assessors,
$n = 5 =$ the number of subjects being ranked.

$$
\begin{aligned}
S_{max} &= \tfrac{1}{12} 4^2 (5^3 - 5) \\
&= 160
\end{aligned}
$$

Kendall's coefficient of concordance is defined as follows and may be calculated:

$$W = \frac{S}{\frac{1}{12}k^2(n^3 - n)} = \frac{106}{160} = 0.663 \qquad (3.4)$$

which is, in reality, the variance of the rank totals as a fraction of the maximum possible variance of the rank totals, that is, if there had been perfect agreement among the assessors. This may be obtained, perhaps more readily, using your calculator. Should you wish to do this, proceed as follows: if there were total agreement between all four assessors, the children A, B, C, D and E would be ranked consistently as 1, 2, 3, 4 and 5, respectively, giving rank totals of 4, 8, 12, 16 and 20. The variance (the square of the standard deviation) of these values may be found with a calculator to be 40. Similarly the variance of the observed rank totals, 5, 10, 14, 12 and 19, may be found to be 26.5. W is given by:

$$W = \frac{\text{Variance of observed rank totals}}{\text{Maximum possible variance of rank totals}} = \frac{26.5}{40}$$
$$= 0.663$$

Thus W may take values between zero, if the rank totals for each child are identical so that the variance is zero, i.e. the ranking is totally at random, and unity in the same way as the positive standard correlation coefficient. The closer the value is to unity, the stronger is the general agreement between the assessors.

The significance of the coefficient may be assessed with reference to Table I in Appendix VI where we can see the critical values of W, for $k = 4$ and $n = 5$, at 5% and 1% significance levels are 0.553 and 0.683 respectively. The observed value of 0.663 is thus significant at the 5% level but not at the 1% level, i.e.

$$0.01 < P < 0.05$$

Remember that this means that the probability that the observed level of agreement has occurred by random chance is greater than 0.01, or 1%, but less than 0.05, or 5%. Thus, if we are prepared to accept up to a 5% chance of being wrong we would reject the null hypothesis (that there is no general agreement) in favour of the alternative that general agreement exists. If, however, we are only prepared to accept a 1% chance of being wrong, we must accept the null hypothesis and conclude that the apparent agreement has occurred by chance.

We should note that this is always a one-way test, i.e. W cannot take negative values, and thus we are assessing a level of general agreement and are unable to draw any conclusion about significant disagreement. If the agreement is not significant, we are only able to conclude that the rankings are assigned at random.

Tied ranks

If the origin of data is in the form of measurements rather than ranks, it is possible that two observations may have the same value, whereupon the ranks will be the same. Tied ranks, such as these, are treated in the usual way by assigning an average rank, for example, the data 6, 7, 7, 9 would be ranked 1, 2.5, 2.5 and 4. As was the case using Spearman's formula for the rank correlation coefficient, the calculation of W is affected by the presence of tied ranks, which have a depressive effect on the value of W. If there are only a few ties and the number of ranks is relatively large, the effect is fairly small; however, if the number of ranks is rather small, the effect can be appreciable and it is advisable to apply a correction.

Unfortunately this situation cannot be remedied quite as simply as in the case of the Spearman rank correlation coefficient, where we can use the Pearson formula (Equation 3.2) for the calculation using the ranks, rather than the values, of the data. The way in which the correction is applied to Kendall's coefficient of concordance is demonstrated in the following example:

Example 3.6

Three sets of data were ranked as follows:

	Ranks					
Data set X	1	5	3.5	3.5	2	6
Y	1.5	1.5	4	4	4	6
Z	2	1	3	4	5	6
Rank totals	4.5	7.5	10.5	11.5	11	18

$$\text{Mean rank total} = M_T = \frac{4.5 + 7.5 + 10.5 + 11.5 + 11 + 18}{6}$$

$$= 10.5$$

$$S = \sum (\text{Rank total} - \text{Mean rank total})^2$$
$$= \sum (R_T - M_T)^2$$
$$= (4.5 - 10.5)^2 + (7.5 - 10.5)^2 + \cdots$$
$$+ (11 - 10.5)^2 + (18 - 10.5)^2$$
$$= 36 + 9 + 0 + 1 + 0.25 + 56.25$$
$$= 102.5$$

$$\tfrac{1}{12}k^2(n^3 - n) = \tfrac{1}{12}3^2(6^3 - 6) = 157.5$$

Thus, without the correction:

$$W = \frac{S}{\tfrac{1}{12}k^2(n^3 - n)} = \frac{102.5}{157.5} = 0.651$$

The correction is applied by calculating the following quantity for each set of rankings:

$$T = \frac{\sum (t^3 - t)}{12}$$

where t is the number of observations tied for a given rank in a particular group. Incorporating the correction the coefficient now becomes:

$$W = \frac{S}{\tfrac{1}{12}k^2(n^3 - n) - k\sum T} \tag{3.5}$$

where:

$$\sum T = T_X + T_Y + T_Z$$

In Group X we have two ranks tied at 3.5, so that $t = 2$:

$$T_x = \frac{\sum (t^3 - t)}{12} = \frac{(2^3 - 2)}{12} = 0.5$$

and in Group Y we have two ranks tied at 1.5 and three ranks tied at 4:

$$T_Y = \frac{\sum (t^3 - t)}{12} = \frac{(2^3 - 2) + (3^3 - 3)}{12} = 2.5$$

and in Group Z there are no tied ranks, therefore:

$$T_Z = 0$$

and

$$\sum T = 0.5 + 2.5 = 3$$

The Kendall coefficient, corrected for tied ranks, may now be calculated (Equation 3.5):

$$W = \frac{102.5}{\frac{1}{12} 3^2 (6^3 - 6) - 3(3)}$$

$$= 0.690$$

Reference to Table I shows that critical value of W at the 5% level for $k = 3$ and $n = 6$ is 0.660. The uncorrected value of 0.651 is therefore not significant, suggesting that there is no general agreement between the assessors, whereas the corrected value of 0.690 is larger than the critical value so that we would conclude that they do, in general, agree with each other.

Linear regression

The *linear regression* procedure, or, as it is sometimes called, the 'method of least squares', is a process by which the 'line of best fit' may be drawn through a series of points when there is evidence to suggest that the relationship is linear. This latter point is very important and a regression should not be applied to the whole range of data if they follow a relationship such as that illustrated in Figure 3.6 which represents the change in weight of an individual following an exercise routine. The relationship appears to be linear up to about the eighth month so it is quite legitimate to regress the limited part of these data up to that point.

The line of best fit represents the most probable values of the dependent variable (y) for given values of the independent variable

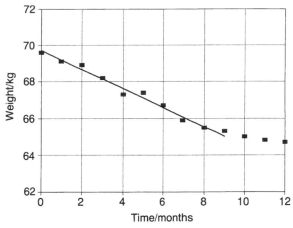

Figure 3.6 *Data showing a linear relationship over a limited part of the range*

(*x*), and the equation describing this line, the *regression equation*, may thus be used to predict the most probable value of the *dependent variable* for any given value of the *independent variable*.

In Figure 3.3 the linear regression line has been included to show the general trend. The procedure will now be considered in more detail.

If a dozen individuals were presented with the scatterplot shown in Figure 3.7a and were asked to draw what appeared to be the best line through the points, most of the lines would be very similar, but each one would be positioned by the subjective assessment of each individual. The linear regression procedure positions the line such that the sum of the squares of the *residuals*, that is the value of $\sum (y - \hat{y})^2$, where y is the observed value, and $\hat{y}$ is the value of y lying on the straight line, or the 'predicted value', are minimized. The squares are taken because some are positive, and some are negative, and thus by taking the square a positive quantity is maintained. The residuals are shown as the vertical lines in Figure 3.7b.

The regression equation

An equation of the form which follows describes a straight line, where A and B are sometimes referred to as the 'regression constants':

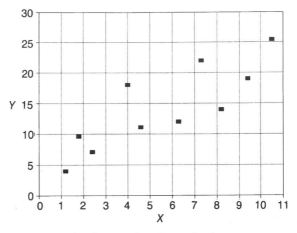

Figure 3.7a *A scatterplot showing the relationship between two sets of data*

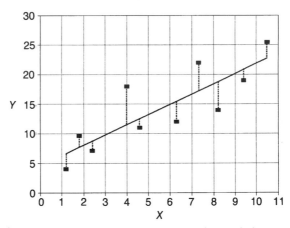

Figure 3.7b *The same data as in Figure 3.7a together with the regression line. The residuals, which are minimized by the regression procedure, are also shown*

$$y = A + Bx$$

where:
B = the slope of the line,
A = the intercept on the y axis when x is zero.

The slope of the line is simply the increase in y for each unit increase in x. Just as a road sign may indicate a '1 in 10' or '10%' hill, which means that you climb up one unit as you move forward ten units.

The slope is thus 1/10 or 0.1. If y decreases as x increases, the slope is negative.

It can be shown that, for the square of the residuals to be a minimum:

$$B = \frac{\sum xy - n\bar{x}\bar{y}}{\sum x^2 - n\bar{x}^2} \tag{3.6}$$

and since the linear equation applies to all pairs of values of x and y, it will also apply to the average value of each, i.e.

$$\bar{y} = A + B\bar{x}$$

which may be rearranged:

$$A = \bar{y} - B\bar{x} \tag{3.7}$$

so that the intercept may also be calculated. Consider the following example:

Example 3.7

It has been suggested that the range of hip movement (Movt) in patients suffering from osteoarthritis is linearly dependent on body weight. In order to test this hypothesis, the following data were collected from ten patients:

Wt (lb)	140	128	170	132	154	135	143	149	158	162
Movt %	40	45	25	40	30	35	45	40	30	25

In this example we shall:

(a) calculate the Pearson correlation coefficient and determine its significance from the appropriate tables;
(b) perform a regression analysis of hip movement on body weight and write the regression equation;
(c) plot a scatter diagram and draw the regression line (the line of best fit) through the points;
(d) estimate the most probable hip movement in a patient who weighs 154 lb.

If a calculator with a linear regression function is not available, then Equations 3.2, 3.6 and 3.7 may be used to obtain the correlation coefficient and the regression constants. Firstly the following quantities are calculated, where x is the independent variable (body weight) and y is the dependent variable (hip movement):

$$\bar{x} = \frac{\sum x}{n} = 147.1 \qquad\qquad \bar{y} = \frac{\sum y}{n} = 35.5$$

$$s_x = 13.84 \qquad\qquad s_y = 7.62$$

$$\sum x^2 = 218,107 \qquad \sum xy = 51,420$$

$$n = 10$$

r may now be calculated:

$$r = \frac{1}{(10-1)} \left(\frac{51,420 - 10(147.1)(35.5)}{(13.86)(7.62)} \right)$$

$$= -0.843$$

Note that, at this stage, it is wise to extract $\sum x^2$ from the calculator because, although not required for the calculation of the correlation coefficient, it is required for the regression constants.

The correlation coefficient indicates a fairly strong negative correlation, i.e. although there is considerable scatter, it can be seen in Figure 3.8 that there is a distinct trend in that the range of movement decreases with increasing body weight, i.e. a negative correlation.

The question then arises: does an increase in body weight cause a decrease in the range of movement? The correlation coefficient indicates that there is a strong negative correlation, that is, the range of movement decreases as the body weight increases, but this does not necessarily mean that the former causes the latter: there is no evidence in the data collected to indicate that an increase in body weight *causes* a reduction in the range of movement. Intuitively, we may feel that this is the case, but the statistical procedure simply tells us that as one increases the other decreases, but says nothing about cause and effect. It is possible that another independent factor affects both of these variables, but in opposite directions.

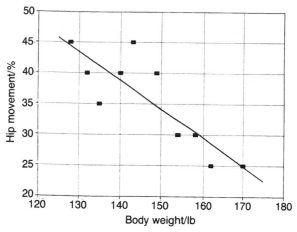

Figure 3.8 *A negative correlation with regression line and residuals*

Referring to the data given above, and to Equations 3.6 and 3.7, the regression constants, A and B, may now be calculated as follows:

$$B = \frac{51,420 - 10(147.1)(35.5)}{218,107 - 10(147.1)^2}$$

$$= -0.4646$$

and

$$A = \bar{y} - Bx$$

$$= 35.5 - (-0.4646)(147.1)$$

$$- 35.5 \mid 68.343$$

$$= 103.8$$

Thus the regression equation may be written:

$$y = 103.8 - 0.465(x)$$

or, rather more explicitly:

$$(\%\ \text{Hip movement}) = 103.8 - 0.465\ (\text{body weight})$$

We should note that this is referred to as 'a regression of percentage hip movement on body weight', or in general, 'a regression of y on x'. The equation, or the regression line on the plot, may be used to predict the most probable percentage hip movement for a given body weight. Once again, however, a little thought is necessary before making predictions, for example, if the body weight is zero, the predicted percentage hip movement is 103.8%, which is clearly nonsense. Similarly, if the body weight was 223.2 lb (15 stone 13 lb, the predicted percentage hip movement is zero, and if heavier than this, it becomes negative. Both of these situations are clearly absurd and emphasize the point that predictions should only be made within the range of the regression, or, perhaps, slightly outside that range.

Having obtained the regression equation, the 'line of best fit' may be drawn on the plot. This is readily achieved by selecting two arbitrary values of x, near the top and bottom of the scale respectively, and calculating the corresponding y values.

For example, if values of body weight (x) of 125 and 175 are taken, the corresponding values of the most probable percentage hip movement, calculated from the regression equation, are 45.7 and 22.4 respectively. The two points $(x = 125, y = 45.7)$ and $(x = 175, y = 22.4)$ may then be placed on the graph and a straight line drawn between them.

It is necessary only to determine the position of two points because all the values of y calculated from the regression equation will, of course, lie on the regression line.

The regression equation gives values for the most probable percentage hip movement for any specified body weight, i.e. for a weight of 154 lb:

$$(\% \text{ Hip movement}) = 103.8 - 0.465(154)$$

$$= 32$$

Note that a value of 30% has been observed for a patient with a body weight of 154 lb. This, however, is a single observation and, considering the data as a whole, we conclude that if many such patients, all with a weight of 154 lb, were observed, the most probable hip movement would be 32%.

Transformation of data

In some instances the relationship between two variables may not be linear, but may be rendered so by a simple transformation, e.g. the y values may be transformed by taking the logarithm, the square, the reciprocal or the square root. This procedure may be a little labour intensive if performed with a hand calculator but is very easily achieved with a statistical package such as MINITAB on a computer. The reason for transformation is that a regression equation to describe a straight line, i.e. a line of best fit, can be determined very much more easily than an equation to fit a curve. Consider the following example:

Example 3.8

The following data represent the growth of a tumour induced in a laboratory animal:

v	0.3	0.6	2.1	2.7	5.8	7.3	9.6	14.4	16.0	23.0	26.2	27.0	34.8	38.4	47.6
t	12	14	16	18	20	22	24	26	28	30	32	34	36	38	40

where v = the volume/ml and t = time/days.

Consider the various transformations illustrated in the plots shown in Figures 3.9 to 3.13. It can be seen that in Figures 3.9 to 3.12, the relationships are clearly not linear, however, the plot of the square root of the volume against time appears to be so and, on performing the regression, the line of best fit may be added as shown. For the regression in this case, of course, x is time and y is $\sqrt{\text{(volume)}}$.

We should remember that regression analysis should not be performed on data when it is possible to see, by looking at the plot, that the relation is not linear, or is perhaps linear over only part of the range.

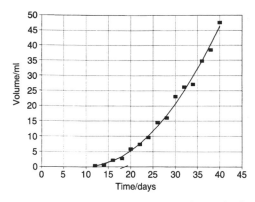

Figure 3.9 *A plot showing the non-linear rate of growth of a tumour*

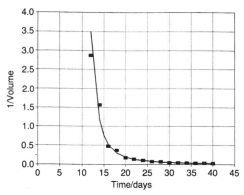

Figure 3.10 *A non-linear plot of the reciprocal of the volume against time*

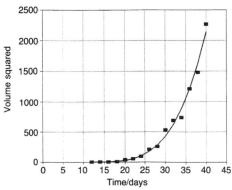

Figure 3.11 *A non-linear plot of the square of the volume against time*

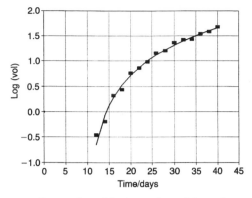

Figure 3.12 *A non-linear plot of the logarithm of the volume against time*

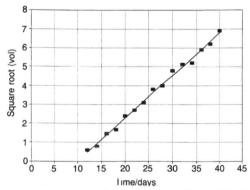

Figure 3.13 *A transformation of the data from Figure 3.9 which results in a linear relationship so that the regression line can be drawn*

Summary

CORRELATION COEFFICIENT (*r*) is a measure of the strength of the linear relationship between observations taken in pairs. If *y* increases as *x* increases, the correlation coefficient is positive; if *y* decreases as *x* increases, it is negative. By definition it may only take values between +1.0 and −1.0. If the correlation is perfect, i.e. the points lie exactly on a straight line, $r = +1.0$, if the slope is positive, and $r = -1.0$ if it is negative.

THE SIGNIFICANCE OF THE CORRELATION COEF-FICIENT is the probability that the observed value could have occurred by chance; this may be determined from tables.

ONE-WAY AND TWO-WAY TESTS. Hypothesis tests may be one-way (directional) or two-way (non-directional) depending on the alternative or experimental hypothesis.

KENDALL'S COEFFICIENT OF CONCORDANCE is a measure of the general agreement in ranking of a number of subjects by several judges or assessors. This is always a one-way test in that the null hypothesis asserts that there is no agreement and the alternative is that the agreement is significant, i.e. it cannot assess disagreement.

LINEAR REGRESSION, sometimes referred to as the method of least squares, is a procedure which produces a regression equation which enables the most probable value of the y variable to be predicted for any given value of the x variable and the line of best fit to be drawn on the scatterplot.

Exercises for Chapter 3

Exercise 3.1

Two speech therapists were tasked to rank five aphasic children in order of ability with the following results:

	Child				
	A	B	C	D	E
Therapist 1	2	3	4	5	1
Therapist 2	2	4	5	3	1

Is there agreement in their assessments?

Exercise 3.2

An occupational therapist used a grip tester with a volunteer patient who had suffered a hand injury and was undertaking an exercise routine. The grip strength was measured twice a week on Mondays and Thursdays with the following results:

Time/days   1   4   8 11 15 18 22 25 29 32 36 39 43

Force/kg   24 28 29 32 37 37 41 43 45 46 45 47 46

(a) Plot the points on a graph.
(b) Calculate the correlation coefficient using (i) all the data and (ii) using only that part which appears to be linearly related.
(c) Determine the regression constants over an appropriate range, write the linear equation, and draw the regression line, or line of best fit, on the plot.

Exercise 3.3

The winning time in the 400 m final in a particular athletics club for ten consecutive years was recorded as follows:

Time/s 50.50 50.00 50.50 49.60 50.05 49.48 49.60 49.00 49.30 48.90

(a) Regress the time on year (year on the x-axis), write the equation, plot the points and draw the line of best fit.
(b) Calculate the correlation coefficient and determine its significance from the tables.
(c) Predict the most probable winning time for the following year and for 20 years after the last recorded time above. Do you think that these are reliable predictions?

Exercise 3.4

Ten students were asked to rank three textbooks in order of preference with the following results:

Student	Textbook I	II	III
A	3	1	2
B	1	3	2
C	3	2	1
D	1	2	3
E	1	3	2
F	2	1	3
G	1	2	3
H	1	3	2
I	3	2	1
J	1	2	3

Is there general agreement in the rating of the three books by the students?

Exercise 3.5

Three different vocabulary tests to assess children with learning and recognition difficulties were compared using a group of six children. Each test comprised ten parts and the number correctly recognized by each child was recorded as follows:

	Child A	B	C	D	E	F	G
Test I	8	6	7	7	10	4	4
Test II	9	9	9	7	5	5	4
Test III	8	10	9	6	6	5	4
Test IV	10	9	9	4	7	7	5

Can it be concluded that the four tests are in general agreement with each other?

4

The Concept of Probability and the Normal Distribution

Contents
—The concept of probability.
—The normal distribution.
—The standard normal distribution tables.

Introduction

The concept of probability, which is crucial in any considerations concerning inferential statistics, was introduced in Chapter 1. Extending the ideas to consider probability distributions is also very important, and the most fundamental of these is the *normal distribution* or, as it is sometimes called, the Gaussian distribution. Such a curve is symmetrical and is often described as 'bell-shaped'.

As a preliminary, it is worth spending a little time considering the nature of probability and probability distributions in general, because we will come across a number of different types as we progress. The following examples involving the tossing of coins have been included because, it is hoped, they will help to give an understanding of the nature of probability and they represent experiments which may easily be performed if desired.

Probability

The development of ideas concerning probability was stimulated by rich gamblers who were anxious to increase their winnings, or perhaps decrease their losses, and so they employed mathematicians, many famous names among them, to assess the merits of particular strategies. Early probability theory has developed into the ideas of inferential statistics, whereby inferences about a whole population may be drawn from data collected from samples, or samples may be compared with each other.

Probability is a very important concept. The term is used in everyday language in a somewhat vague way, for example:

'It will probably rain today'.
'If this wind does not stop, my garden fence will probably be blown down.'

These statements are not at all quantitative, although we all know that they mean the events described are likely to occur, whatever that may mean. Inferential statistics is concerned with attempting to quantify such probabilities. In some cases this may be done absolutely, sometimes known as an 'a priori' probability, i.e. it can be calculated in advance and is not dependent on experience, for example, the probability of obtaining any particular number when rolling a die. Since there are six faces on a cube and only one of them displays a 'four', the probability of obtaining that 'four' is 1 in 6, 1/6 or 0.167. Thus if a die is rolled 60 times, the 'expected' number of occasions in which 'four' will be obtained is 10, i.e. $(1/6) \times 60$, although in practice this may well not be the case. However, if this 'experiment' (rolling the die 60 times) is repeated a very large number of times, the average number of 'fours' obtained will be 10. The histogram in Figure 4.1 displays the probability, which has been calculated mathematically, of any particular number of occurrences of, say, 'four', when the die is rolled 60 times.

We can see that the probability of obtaining either 2 or 20 fours in 60 throws is very small, and the probability of obtaining fewer than 2, or more than 20, can be seen to be virtually zero, i.e. these are exceedingly unlikely events. We can also see that the most probable event is that 10 fours will be obtained, although the probabilities of obtaining 8, 9, 10 or 11 are not very different.

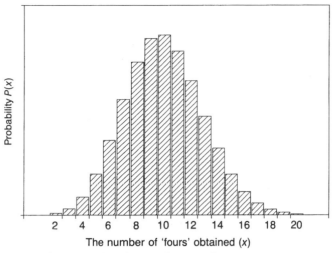

Figure 4.1 *A frequency distribution showing the expected number of 'fours' that would be obtained when a die is rolled 60 times. The distribution is not quite symmetrical because the probability of obtaining a four in a single throw is 1/6 (0.167) rather than 1/2 (0.5)*

If the die is rolled a very large number of times, say 6 million, then the number of 'fours' obtained would be very close to 1 million, i.e. we would expect to obtain 1 million 'ones', 1 million 'twos', 1 million 'threes', etc.

The tree diagram

If we consider the tossing of a coin, it is evident that there are two possible outcomes, i.e. a head or a tail. If we consider the probability of obtaining a head, then, clearly, there is only one favourable outcome, so that the probability of this event occurring is 1/2 or 0.5. The probability of obtaining a given number of heads in tossing several coins (or, of course, several tosses of a single coin) may be seen in a 'tree diagram'.

Outcomes when tossing two coins—a tree diagram

If we consider firstly the simple case of two tosses, the possible outcomes are shown in Figure 4.2. A point worth stressing is that the

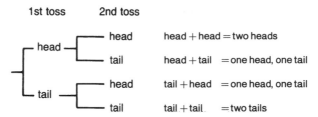

Figure 4.2 *A tree diagram showing the possible outcomes of tossing a coin twice*

probability of obtaining a head with a single toss is constant at 0.5, i.e. each toss is independent and is not influenced by the result of a previous toss. It is sometimes mistakenly believed that if we toss a coin five times and obtain a head each time, the probability of obtaining a head on the sixth toss is greater than 0.5. This is not so, the probability is still 0.5, provided, of course, that we have a normal well-balanced coin.

As far as the result after two tosses is concerned, an outcome yielding a head followed by a tail is equivalent to one in which a tail is followed by a head, i.e. one of each. We can see from the tree diagram that four different outcomes are possible, one with two heads, two with one of each, and one with two tails. Thus the probability of obtaining two heads is 0.25 or 1/4, one head is 0.5 or 2/4, and no heads 0.25 or 1/4. This means that if the experiment (i.e. tossing the coin twice) is conducted, say 12 times, there will be, of course, only one of the four possible outcomes in each case, and in the 12 experiments the 'expected' number of outcomes showing two heads is $0.25 \times 12 = 3$, one head $0.5 \times 12 = 6$, and no heads $0.25 \times 12 = 3$. Remember that these are the 'expected' values; we would not be very surprised, if, with only 12 experiments, we did not find this to be so.

Outcomes from a very large number of experiments

If, however, the experiment were to be conducted very many times, say 1 million, then the number of occasions in which two heads, one head and no heads, respectively, would be observed would be very close to 250,000, 500,000 and 250,000. That is to say, observed values are predicted closely by probabilities only when very large numbers are involved.

Outcomes when tossing three coins

The above considerations may readily be extended to the tossing of three or more coins. We see in Figure 4.3 that in the case of three tosses, there are two possible outcomes from each toss and eight possible from each experiment. As before, we are not concerned with the order in which they occur, only with the final numbers, so that, for example, the results HHT, HTH and THH are all equivalent. Thus a final outcome of two heads and a tail from three tosses has a probability of 3/8, or 0.375. Consequently all the probabilities are:

$$P(3 \text{ heads}) = 1/8 = 0.125$$
$$P(2 \text{ heads}, 1 \text{ tail}) = 3/8 = 0.375$$
$$P(1 \text{ heads}, 2 \text{ tail}) = 3/8 = 0.375$$
$$P(3 \text{ tails}) = 1/8 = 0.125$$

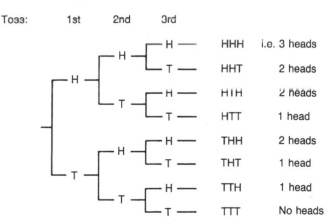

Figure 4.3 *A tree diagram showing the possible outcomes of tossing a coin three times*

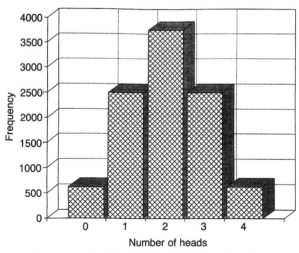

Figure 4.4 *A frequency distribution showing the results of 10,000 experiments of tossing a coin four times*

You may care to construct a similar diagram to represent four tosses of the coin, whereupon it will be found that there are 16 possible outcomes and the respective probabilities of obtaining 4, 3, 2, 1 and zero heads are 1/16, 4/16, 6/16, 4/16 and 1/16. If the experiment in this case were to be conducted, say, 10,000 times, then the expected frequency with which each outcome would be observed is given by the probability multiplied by the total number of experiments, i.e. 625, 2,500, 3,750, 2,500 and 625 respectively. So that in 625 occasions, four heads would be expected, in 2,500 occasions three heads and one tail, and so on.

The result may be represented as a histogram if desired, with either the probability or the frequency displayed against the number of heads obtained, as in Figure 4.4, which shows clearly that the distribution is symmetrical.

Outcomes when tossing 30 coins

If the number of tosses is increased to, say, 30, a tree diagram could still be drawn, but would require a very large piece of paper and

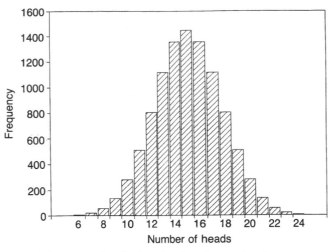

Figure 4.5 *A frequency distribution showing the results of 10,000 experiments of tossing a coin 30 times*

would be exceedingly tedious. Fortunately there are easier ways of obtaining these probabilities, namely by referring to the binomial distribution, although it is not necessary to consider this here. Looking at the above examples, a little thought will show that, because there are two possible outcomes from each toss, the total possible number for three tosses is $2 \times 2 \times 2$, or 2^3, so that for n tosses, the number is 2^n. Thus, for 30 tosses of the coin there are $2^{30} = 1,073,741,824$ possible outcomes, which is, perhaps, a little difficult to believe. As before, the probability of each of these outcomes is the same, and, of course, many of them will be equivalent because we are only concerned with the number of heads and tails and not the order in which they arise. For example, there are 30 different ways of arriving at 1 head and 29 tails, and it can be shown that 15 heads and 15 tails can arise in 155,117,520 different ways.

If the experiment (tossing a coin 30 times) is repeated 10,000 times and the number of heads obtained in each experiment is recorded, the results, if displayed in a histogram, would look like Figure 4.5. We can see that the outline of the histogram is becoming close to a smooth curve and sets of data, where the variability is the result of random factors, will follow such a symmetrical curve which is said to be a *normal distribution*. This particular curve is symmetrical because the probability of obtaining a head is equal to the probability of not obtaining a head, i.e. the probability of obtaining a tail.

Referring back to the example shown in Figure 4.1, where the data results from rolling a die 60 times, we can see that the histogram is not quite symmetrical. This is because the probability of obtaining a 'four' is not 0.5, but 1/6, i.e. 0.167, thus the distribution is a little heavier on the left and 'skewed' to the right.

In the above examples we are concerned with *discrete data*, that is, we are counting objects, people or events, in this case the number of heads obtained. However, if we consider *continuous data* where measurements are taken and the number of decimal places is determined only by the instrument which is employed for the purpose, then in order to construct a histogram, the observations or measurements are divided into 'classes' or 'groups' (see Chapter 2).

Referring to Figure 2.4 in Chapter 2, we see what we can readily accept to be a symmetrical distribution, and the frequency with which observations fall within any particular class, divided by the total number of observations, is a measure of the probability of that class. For example, there is a total of 250 observations, and 31 of these fall within the class 34–35 inches, so we can estimate that the probability that a person chosen at random would have a chest girth within this range is 31/250 = 0.124, i.e. the probability is represented by the area of that class as a fraction of the total area. Similarly, the probability that the girth would lie within the range 34–38 inches is the area of the four central classes as a fraction of the whole, i.e. $(31 + 37 + 42 + 30)/250 = 0.56$.

If we accept that our sample of 250 is a reasonable representation of the population of male students as a whole, we would conclude that 56% of all male students would have a chest girth between 34 and 38 inches.

An important principle

The area under a probability distribution curve between specific limits is a measure of the probability of an observation falling between those limits.

The normal distribution

As we have seen from the above, the normal distribution is bell-shaped and symmetrical, and most observations are close to the mean, which is at the centre, becoming less frequent as values become remote from the mean.

Consider a population with a normal distribution which has a mean of 50 and a standard deviation of 5. If a large number of measurements was taken and the data grouped into classes with a class width of 1.0, a histogram, as in Figure 4.6, may be drawn. The distribution is symmetrical about the mean and the probability that a measurement will fall into any particular class is given by the area of that class as a fraction of the total area.

If the width of a class were reduced to, say, 0.5, the probability of that class will clearly be reduced because its area becomes a smaller fraction of the whole. Thus the probability of each class becomes smaller as the width decreases so that the ratio, which is usually called the *probability density function* (PDF), is defined:

$$\text{PDF} = \frac{\text{Probability of a class}}{\text{Width of the class}}$$

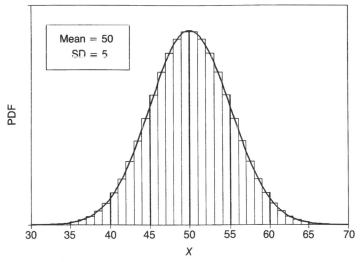

Figure 4.6 *A histogram representing a large amount of data which follows a normal distribution with a mean of 50 and a standard deviation of 5*

Both the 'probability of a class' and the 'width of the class' tend to zero as a larger number of classes is taken, but the ratio remains finite, so that in the limit, when the classes are infinitely narrow, we have a smooth curve and the vertical axis represents the probability density function.

We have seen above that the area under the probability distribution curve between any given limits is a measure of the probability that an observation or measurement will fall between those limits. For any given set of data, where the population mean and standard deviation are known, a set of statistical tables could be prepared giving the area under the curve for various values of x, thus enabling the relevant probabilities to be calculated. The tables, however, would then apply only to that set of data which has the given mean and standard deviation and, to cover all eventualities, it would be necessary to have an infinite number of sets of tables. This clearly is not feasible. The problem is overcome by using a *standard normal distribution* as follows.

The standard normal distribution

The 'standard normal distribution' is one in which the differences between each observation (x) and the mean (μ) are represented in units of standard deviation and given the symbol Z, so that the same sets of tables may be used for *any* data.

Thus, for example, if x is 2 standard deviations greater than the mean, $Z = +2.0$, if x is 1.5 standard deviations below the mean, $Z = -1.5$, and so on. Z is therefore defined:

$$Z = \frac{x - \mu}{\sigma} \tag{4.1}$$

When $Z = $ zero, the observation x is equal to the mean, and when $Z = +1.0$, x is 1 standard deviation from the mean, thus the standard normal distribution is one with the mean at 0 and a standard deviation of unity.

The vertical axis displays the *probability density function* or PDF, which, although not strictly correct, may be looked upon as a measure of the relative probabilities or frequencies with which

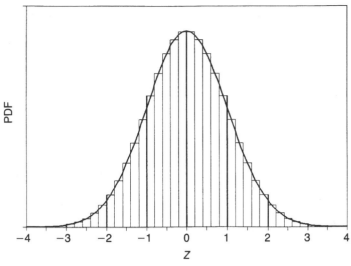

Figure 4.7 *A standard normal distribution where the mean is zero and the standard deviation is unity. In this distribution, deviations from the mean are represented in units of standard deviation*

observations of any particular value of Z would be expected to occur. In addition, the total area under the curve has been adjusted so that it is equal to unity and, therefore, the area between any two points is a direct measure of the probability that Z will fall between these two values by chance. This is, of course, the same as saying that this is the probability that a value of x will fall between the two values which correspond to the two Z values.

This means that if we make a large number of observations or measurements on members of a given population, we can calculate the 'Z-score', that is the value of Z for each measurement, and by placing them in the appropriate class prepare a histogram. If we have an exceedingly large number of observations and the class width is narrow enough, the outline of the histogram will approach a smooth normal distribution, with zero mean and unit standard deviation. Such a situation is shown in Figure 4.7, which, you will see, is identical to Figure 4.6 except the observations are represented in units of standard deviation, rather than the units of measurement.

Statistical tables showing the area under the curve to the left of any given value of Z, which indicates the probability that a value of Z less than that value will occur by chance if Z is zero, are given in

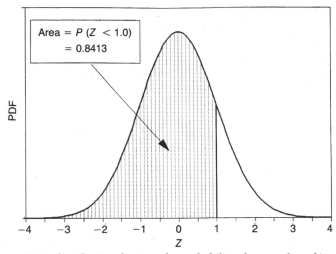

Area = P (Z < 1.0)
     = 0.8413

Figure 4.8 *A distribution showing the probability that a value of Z will be observed below unity, i.e. a value of the variable which is less than one standard deviation above the mean*

Table A in Appendix VI. The area corresponding to this probability is often referred to as the *cumulative density function* (CDF) because it is a measure of the cumulative probability density up to that value of Z.

An example may be seen in Figure 4.8 which shows the probability that Z will take a value below unity, including any negative value. This presupposes, of course, that the data follows a normal distribution.

Warning

Unfortunately the symbols used in statistics vary to some extent between texts and what is referred to as Z above (the most common symbol), is sometimes called '*d*', '*u*' or even '*x*'. The latter, which is used in the *Cambridge Elementary Statistical Tables*, may lead to confusion since *x* is the symbol usually used for the 'random variable', i.e. the value of the observation or measurement.

In addition statistical tables are not always printed in the same form. Some tables, such as Table A, give the area to the left of Z, i.e. the CDF (cumulative density function), which is sometimes referred to as $\phi(Z)$, for example, the area to the left of $Z = 0.75$, which represents the probability that $Z < 0.75$, would be written $\phi(0.75)$. In some publications, the tables give the value in the tail to the right of Z, and others give the area between $Z = 0$ and Z, which is often referred to as $A(Z)$. Thus it is important to be quite clear what is being represented when tables are consulted.

Example 4.1

What is the probability that Z will exceed unity, i.e. a value of x more than 1.0 standard deviation above the mean will be observed?

If we refer to Table A, we find that if $Z = 1.0$, the tabulated probability, the CDF, or $\phi(1.0)$, which we should remember, refers to the probability that a value of Z will occur below 1.0, is 0.8413 (see Figure 4.8), which means that the probability that Z will exceed this value is $(1 - 0.8413) = 0.1587$.

Negative values of Z

Negative values of Z are usually not included in tables because the distribution is symmetrical. For example, the area to the left of, say, $Z = -0.5$, is exactly the same as the area to the right of $Z = +0.5$.

Also we should note that, in the case of a continuous distribution such as this, there is no distinction between 'the probability that Z is greater than 1.0' and 'the probability that Z is greater than or equal to 1.0'. This is because the probability that Z will be exactly equal to 1.0, i.e. 1.000 000 . . . with as many zeros as one cares to add, becomes, in the limit, zero.

Thus, for *any* set of data which follows a normal distribution, the probability that an observation or measurement will be greater than one standard deviation above the mean is 0.1587, i.e. we would expect 15.87% of the observations to be equal to, or greater than, one standard deviation above the mean. In addition, since the distribution is symmetrical, 15.87% of the observations would be less than one standard deviation below the mean. Thus, within the

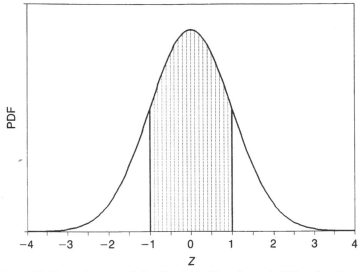

Figure 4.9 *From the normal distribution tables, the probability that Z < 1.0 is 0.8413 (see also Figure 4.8), thus the probability that Z > 1.0 is (1 − 0.8413) = 0.1587, which, because of the symmetry of the distribution, is the same as the probability that Z < −1.0. Therefore the probability that Z will be between −1.0 and +1.0 is given by (0.8413 − 0.1587) = 0.6826*

range $\mu \pm \sigma$ we would find $100 - (2 \times 15.87)\%$, i.e. 68.26%, as shown in Figure 4.9.

In a similar way, other ranges can be determined, and it is useful to note that the following percentages of the observations would be expected to fall within the limits shown:

$$\mu \pm \sigma = 68.26\%$$

$$\mu \pm 2\sigma = 95.46\%$$

$$\mu \pm 3\sigma = 99.73\%$$

Reference to Figure 4.10 shows the limits outside of which 5% of observations would be expected to fall in a normal distribution, i.e. $\mu \pm 1.96\sigma$, which is, of course, very close to $\mu \pm 2\sigma$, which is often taken as an approximation.

These limits, and similar limits for other distributions, are very important in the context of statistical inference and significance, and are considered in Chapter 5.

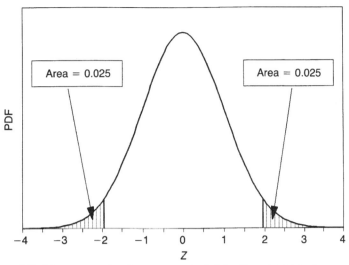

Figure 4.10 *The area under the curve excluded by* $Z = \pm1.96$ *is shown and can be seen to be* $(2 \times 0.025) = 0.05$ *or* 5%

Example 4.3

If the mean and standard deviation resting pulse rate of the population at large are 72 and 8 respectively, what percentage of the population would be expected to have a resting pulse rate above 80?

$$Z = \frac{x - \mu}{\sigma}$$
$$= \frac{80 - 72}{8} = 1.0$$

Referring to Table A, we can see that when $Z = 1.0$, the area to the left of Z, the cumulative density function (CDF), or $\phi(Z)$, which in this case would be written $\phi(1.0)$, is 0.8413. This is the probability that, if a person is chosen at random from the population, Z will be less than 1.0, or in this case, since $\mu = 72$ and $\sigma = 8$, x will be less than 80, i.e.

$$P(Z < 1.0) = P(x < 80) = 0.8413$$

However, we require the probability that x is greater than 80. So, as in Example 4.1, since the total probability is unity:

$$P(Z > 1.0) = P(x > 80) = 1 - P(x < 80)$$
$$= 1 - 0.8413$$
$$= 0.1587$$

Thus the probability that a person chosen at random will have a resting pulse rate greater than 80 is 0.1587. If 100 people are chosen at random we would expect 15.87 of them to have such a pulse rate. We obviously cannot have 0.87 of a person, but what this means is that if we selected many samples of 100 persons, the average number having a pulse rate over 80 would be 15.87. We can conclude, therefore, that about 16% of the population as a whole would be expected to have a resting pulse rate greater than 80.

The inverse cumulative density function

We have seen that, provided the data follows a normal distribution, the cumulative density function (CDF) represents the probability that an observation will be found below any given value of Z. Should we require to consider the reverse situation, that is, to determine the value of Z below which we would expect, say, 90% of observations to be found, we need to look in the body of the normal distribution tables (Table A) for 0.90. This is because, of course, we require the value of Z *below* which the probability of an observation occurring is 0.90, or 90%. This is sometimes referred to as the 'inverse cumulative density function' (INVCDF), i.e. INVCDF(0.90). Referring to Table A we find:

Z	$\phi(Z)$
1.28	0.8997
1.29	0.9015

Thus the CDF for $Z = 1.28$ is the closest value to 0.90.

An alternative approach to finding the INVCDF is to refer to the t-distribution tables (Table B in Appendix VI) at an infinite number of degrees of freedom. The t-distribution, which is discussed in Chapter 6, is very similar to the normal distribution except that allowance has been made for the small sample size, or, more strictly, the number of degrees of freedom, and as a consequence it is not feasible to prepare tables covering all values of t for all possible sample sizes, so only the *critical values* are included. However, the larger the sample size, the closer the two distributions become, and when the number of degrees of freedom is infinite, they become identical. Thus the critical values of the normal distribution, i.e. values of Z for the exclusion of specified probabilities in the 'tail' of the distribution may be found from the t-distribution tables when the number of degrees of freedom is infinite. For percentages which are not included in the t-distribution table, we must resort to the method described above.

Example 4.2

Assume that the mean systolic blood pressure of 25-year-old males has been estimated at 128 mmHg with a standard deviation of 8 mmHg. What is the value above which 25% of the population would be expected to be found?

Let us consider this example using both of the approaches mentioned above.

Firstly, by reference to the normal distribution tables (Table A).

(a) We require the value of Z which excludes 25% to the right, and, of course, 75% to the left. We therefore need to seek 0.75 in the body of the table. The two values closest to this are:

Z	$\phi(Z)$
0.67	0.7486
0.68	0.7517

Either of these values of Z may be used, there is very little difference in the final result, e.g.

$$Z = \frac{x - \mu}{\sigma}$$

$$\therefore \quad x = \mu + Z\sigma$$

$$= 128 + (0.67)(8)$$

$$= 133.4 \text{ mmHg}$$

(b) Alternatively, using the second approach, if we consult the t-distribution for an infinite number of degrees of freedom:

$$t_{0.25}(df = \infty) = Z = 0.6745$$

$$= \frac{x - \mu}{\sigma}$$

$$\therefore \quad x = \mu + Z\sigma$$

$$= 128 + (0.6745)(8)$$

$$= 133.4 \text{ mmHg}$$

Which, of course, yields the same result.

Summary

PROBABILITY of a final outcome may be obtained from the probabilities of each 'trial' using a tree diagram.

THE NORMAL DISTRIBUTION is bell-shaped and symmetrical and it is found that many sets of data which are subject to random factors follow this distribution.

THE STANDARD NORMAL DISTRIBUTION has been adjusted to have a mean of zero and a standard deviation of unity. Thus deviations from the mean are represented in units of standard deviation so that a single set of tables may be used with any set of data. The Z-score for a particular measurement is the difference between the measurement and the mean expressed in units of standard deviation. For any set of data which follows a normal distribution, the percentage of observations falling, for example, between the mean plus or minus one standard deviation is the same, namely 68.26%.

THE CUMULATIVE DENSITY FUNCTION (CDF) is the quantity which is usually given in normal distribution tables and represents the area under the curve to the left of the given value of Z, or the probability that Z will be less than this value. The area under the standardized distribution curve between given limits represents the probability that an observation or measurement taken at random will fall within those limits.

INVERSE CUMULATIVE DENSITY FUNCTION is the reverse of the CDF, in other words the value of Z for which a specified percentage of the distribution is excluded.

NEGATIVE VALUES FOR Z are usually not quoted but because the distribution is symmetrical, it is not necessary because the probability that Z will exceed, say 1.0, is exactly the same as the probability that Z will be less than −1.0.

Exercises for Chapter 4

Exercise 4.1

During the past year, a manufacturer has produced 15,600 exercise machines. Of these, 785 were returned within the first year for repair. What is the probability that a machine chosen at random will operate for a year without the need for repair?

Exercise 4.2

Assume that the mean and standard deviation resting pulse rates of the population are 72 and 8 per minute, respectively.

(a) What is the probability that a person chosen at random will have a resting pulse rate between 65 and 85?
(b) In a group of 625 people, how many would be expected to have a pulse rate within that range?

Exercise 4.3

Consider a normal population with mean 65 and standard deviation 7. Calculate the probability that:

(a)   an observation will exceed (i) 70, (ii) 80, (iii) 45, and (iv) 65;
(b)   an observation will be less than (i) 50, (ii) 68, (iii) 60;
(c)   an observation will fall between (i) 60 and 70, (ii) 50 and 75.

Exercise 4.4

The mean protein concentration in the blood of a large number of apparently healthy individuals was found to be 69 g/l with a standard deviation of 4.5 g/l.

(a)   Estimate the 'reference range', i.e. the range which would be expected to include 95% of the healthy population?
(b)   What percentage of the population would be expected to have a concentration of less than 60 g/l?
(c)   Estimate the interquartile range (the range which includes the middle 50% of the observations).

Exercise 4.5

In an experiment to obtain a norm for a grip test, a large number of adult males between the age of 25 to 30 years were tested and it was found that the mean was 36 kg with standard deviation of 4.2 kg measurement.

(a)   Estimate the reference range.
(b)   Estimate the interquartile range.

Statistical Inference and Significance

Contents
—Introduction to statistical inference.
—Statistical significance.
—The Z-test.
—The P-value and levels of confidence.
—One- and two-way tests.

Introduction

It was indicated in Chapter 1 that, in general, statistics may be separated into the categories of descriptive and inferential. If we were able to collect data on a whole population, inferential statistics would not be necessary. Normally, of course, this is not feasible, it is either impossible because the extent of the population is unknown, or it is simply impractical, because the population is so large.

To come to conclusions regarding a population, therefore, data are collected from a sample. One of the associated problems is to ensure that the sample is representative of the population, i.e. it is a *random* sample.

By definition, such a sample is one in which every member of the population has an equal chance of being included. This clearly presents considerable difficulties and in many cases assumptions are made regarding the randomness of a sample which may, or may not, be justified. Further discussion of random sampling is beyond the scope of this text and all considerations regarding inferences drawn from sample data will assume such samples to be random subsets of the population.

Biological variation and random error

The need to collect data from a sample, or a population if that is feasible, arises because each member of the population is not identical. For example, if measurements are made of, say, the vital lung capacity of a number of different individuals, all of whom are assumed to belong to the same population—for example, they are all male subjects between the ages of 20 and 25 years—we would not expect them all to be exactly the same, i.e. we would observe biological variation. We would, however, expect them to follow a normal distribution because it is found that most natural variables of this kind do so.

In addition, variability will exist as a result of *random error*. For example, if repeated measurements of the vital lung capacity of the same person were taken they would not all be identical because of the variability resulting from random effects over which we have no control. This variation, also, will follow a normal distribution. In this latter case, the population would be represented by the total possible number of replicate measurements that could have been made, which, in principle, is infinite.

It would be hoped that by comparison the random error is much smaller than the biological variation, because when collecting data for the purpose of investigating the variation of a particular property, e.g. height, weight, strength, vital lung capacity, etc., in a population, it is often disregarded, or perhaps recognized only to the extent that the mean of two or three measurements is accepted as the value for that particular individual.

We should note that in such cases, the population may be defined in many different ways, for example, all the healthy individuals in the country, or, perhaps, all those with a particular ethnic background, or of a particular sex, or suffering from a specific disease, e.g. diabetes, in which case a further distinction is possible, i.e. insulin dependent and non-insulin dependent diabetes.

Before we consider statistical inference an additional statistic should be defined.

The standard error of the mean

If a number of samples of size n are taken from a normal population with mean μ and standard deviation σ, it can be shown that the means of those samples will also follow a normal distribution with mean μ, but the standard deviation of those means, usually called the *standard error of the mean*, will be $\sigma/\sqrt{n}$.

Example 5.1

Let us assume, as in Chapter 4, that the mean and standard deviation resting pulse rates in a healthy population are 72 and 8 respectively. If we select at random a large number of separate samples of, say, five individuals from that population and measure the mean of each sample, then the sample means will follow a normal distribution (with mean 72) and the standard error of the mean (standard deviation of the mean) will be $8/\sqrt{5}$, i.e. 3.58. For larger sample sizes of 10 and 50, this becomes 2.53 and 1.13 respectively. This is, of course, what we would expect, that is, as the samples get larger, the variation in their means becomes smaller, and, if the samples are as large as 250, then the standard error is reduced to 0.51.

Remembering, from Chapter 4, that 95% of observations will fall between $\mu \pm 1.96\sigma$, and therefore, in the case of the sample means, 95% will fall between $\mu \pm 1.96(\sigma/\sqrt{n})$, it can be seen that if a large number of samples is taken, the result is as follows.

Sample size	Range including 95% of sample means to the nearest whole number
5	$72 \pm 1.96(8/\sqrt{5})$, or 65 to 79
10	$72 \pm 1.96(8/\sqrt{10})$, or 67 to 77
50	$72 \pm 1.96(8/\sqrt{50})$, or 70 to 74
250	$72 \pm 1.96(8/\sqrt{250})$, or 71 to 73

Statistical inference and significance

We first met the concept of significance in Chapter 3 when looking at the correlation coefficient. The principles involved in the determination of statistical significance are, in general, the same, no matter which distribution is involved. Consider the following simple example.

Example 5.2

Let us assume, once again, that the mean and standard deviation pulse rates in a healthy population are 72 and 8 respectively, and, for simplicity, that the standard deviation of the sample may be taken to be the same as the population. A sample of 40 patients suffering from a particular ailment was found to have a mean resting pulse rate of 76.1. Can it be said that a raised pulse rate is characteristic of this disease?

The argument is as follows.

(a) We calculate, using the standard normal distribution tables, the probability that the observed result would occur *if* the true mean is 72, i.e. that a sample of size 40 will have a mean of 76.1 or larger, the difference being the result of random variation. We are concerned only with the probability that the sample mean will be *greater than* the population mean by this amount so we conduct a one-way test.

(b) If this probability is high, we assume that the difference *is* the result of random variation and the true mean could well be 72.

(c) If the probability is low, i.e. it is very unlikely that the observed
value is the result of random variation, we assume that there
really is a difference, or, in statistical terms, the difference is
'significant'.
(d) The most common criterion, as was the case in Chapter 3 when
we considered the correlation coefficient, is to take the difference to be significant if the probability that it has occurred by
chance is smaller than 5%, or 0.05.

Let us now consider the problem. You will recall that in Chapter 4,
Z was defined:

$$Z = \frac{x - \mu}{\sigma} \tag{5.1}$$

i.e. it represents the number of standard deviations between the
random variable (the observation) and the parameter with which it
is being compared, in this case the population mean, μ.
    The definition may be generalized:

$$Z = \frac{(\text{Random variable}) - (\text{Population parameter})}{\text{SE (Random variable)}} \tag{5.2}$$

If the random variable is a sample mean, the standard deviation
becomes the standard error of the mean, i.e. $\sigma/\sqrt{n}$, which in this
case is $8/\sqrt{40} = 1.265$. Thus the observed sample mean, being 4.1
beats above the population mean, is 3.24 standard errors of the
mean above the population mean. Or, calculating Z rather more
formally:

$$z = \frac{\bar{x} - \mu}{\sigma/\sqrt{n}}$$

$$= \frac{(76.1 \quad 72)}{8/\sqrt{40}}$$

$$= 3.24 \tag{5.3}$$

Reference to Table A of the normal distribution tells us that $\phi(3.24)$,
or the 'cumulative density function' (CDF) for a value of Z of 3.24,
is 0.9994. This is the probability that Z will take this value, or
smaller, by random chance alone. Thus, the probability that a value
of Z larger than 3.24 would occur is $(1 - 0.9994) = 0.0006$, or
0.06%, i.e. it is exceedingly unlikely.

Remember, as was pointed out in Chapter 4, that for a continuous distribution such as the normal, there is no distinction between the 'probability that Z will be equal to, or larger than 3.24' and the 'probability that Z will be larger than 3.24'.

Also, we should note that although the above result is very highly significant from a statistical point of view, it is certainly not from a diagnostic point of view. We can calculate, in a similar manner to Example 4.1, the percentage of the population at large which would be expected to have a resting pulse rate of more than 76.1. Note that the standard deviation for that population, i.e. 8, is used, rather than the standard error of the mean, because here we are concerned with the pulse rate of individuals rather than the mean of a sample, i.e.

$$Z = \frac{(76.1 - 72)}{8} = 0.513$$

Reference to Table A shows that the probability that Z will exceed this value is $1 - 0.7019$, or 0.2981, i.e. the probability that a person chosen at random from the population at large will have a resting pulse rate of at least 76.1 is 0.2981, so that 29.81%, or about 30%, of that healthy population will have such a pulse rate.

Statistical hypotheses

The above considerations are usually encompassed in 'statistical hypotheses' which, for the above example, would be as follows.

The null hypothesis

In general, we start with the *null hypothesis*, which is given the symbol H_0, in which we hypothesize that, as the name suggests, there is no difference between the mean of the population from which the sample was taken and the mean of the specified population. The null hypothesis in this example is represented as:

$$H_0: \ \mu = \mu_0 \quad \text{or} \quad H_0: \ \mu = 72$$

where μ is the mean of the population from which the sample was taken and μ_0 is the mean of the specified population, i.e. 72 in the example above.

The alternative or experimental hypothesis

In Example 5.2, this hypothesis would be represented as:

$$H_1: \ \mu > \mu_0 \quad \text{or} \quad H_0: \ \mu > 72$$

The reason for this is that we are hypothesizing that these patients suffering from this particular disease have a resting pulse rate *higher* than the healthy population. Remember that μ is the mean resting pulse rate for the population from which the sample was taken.

The general principle of this approach is to look for evidence to reject the null hypothesis in favour of the alternative, and if insufficient evidence is found, the null hypothesis is, by default, accepted.

Such evidence is obtained by considering the probability that the observed result would occur if H_0 is true. As was seen above, the probability that Z would take a value of 3.24, or larger, is 0.0006, which is, of course, the probability that the observed value of 76.1, or larger, would be observed for the sample mean as the result of random variation, if the true mean is 72. Since this is very small and a good deal less than the chosen significance level of 5%, or 0.05, the null hypothesis can be rejected in favour of the alternative, so we would conclude that the mean of the sample is greater than 72.

Levels of significance

The level of significance employed when conducting a statistical test should normally be chosen before the test is carried out. It should be emphasized that it represents the risk that you are prepared to take of wrongly rejecting the null hypothesis in favour of the experimental hypothesis. This is, of course, because it represents the probability that the observed result is simply a matter of chance.

The significance level, represented as a probability, is often given the symbol α, so that at the 5% level, $\alpha = 0.05$. The choice is arbitrary, but experience has suggested that 5% is about right for most purposes. It may, perhaps, be a little confusing to see probabilities represented as percentages and also as simple probabilities, but unfortunately this is common practice.

Instinctively, one might feel that if a lower level of significance is chosen, e.g. 1% ($\alpha = 0.01$), then we can be more sure of our result, but if this were done, we would find that the null hypothesis is too often accepted when it would be perfectly legitimate to reject it. Conversely, if a higher level, say 20%, is chosen, the null hypothesis would be rejected in favour of the experimental hypothesis when there really is insufficient evidence to indicate that a real difference exists.

The P-value and level of confidence

The probability of 0.0006 considered above is referred to as the 'P-value', and would be represented as $P = 0.0006$. It is, in general, much better to quote a value for P, rather than having chosen a level of significance of, say, 5%, to simply report that 'the difference (between the means being compared) is significant at 5%', i.e. $P = 0.05$, because this makes no distinction between a result where, for example, $P = 0.045$, when one would perhaps be a little cautious before rejecting H_0, and, as above, when $P = 0.0006$, which is very much less than 0.05.

Indeed, we can reject the null hypothesis with very little chance that we are wrong, in fact, we have 99.94% confidence that we are correct—because the probability that a mean of 76.1, or greater, would be observed by chance is only 0.06%; thus if we reject the null hypothesis there is, at most, only a 0.06% chance that we are wrong, or at least a 99.94% chance that we are right.

The Z-test

A test employing the normal distribution is known as a Z-test, and in order to use such a test, the standard deviation of the population must be known. In most circumstances this is unlikely, although it is generally assumed that if the sample contains at least 30 observations, the standard deviation estimated from that sample may be taken to be a good estimate of the population value and may be used in the Z-test. However, the *t*-test, which is considered in Chapter 6, is designed for small samples and the *t*-distribution, which is similar to the normal distribution but is dependent on sample size, is employed and there seems to be little point in making the approximation to the normal distribution in this case. The Z-test is considered here by way of introduction to the use of statistical tables and because of the overall importance of the normal distribution. In order to conduct a *t*-test, the assumption is made that the data follows, at least approximately, a normal distribution.

From the normal distribution tables, it is possible to obtain a specific value of *P* corresponding to a given value of Z. We will see later that for other distributions, e.g. the *t*-distribution mentioned above, this is, in general, not possible from the tables because other factors, such as the size of the sample, have to be taken into account, so that a very large number of sets of tables would be required. For this reason they are usually restricted and represented in the form of *critical values* or *percentage points*.

It was pointed out in Chapter 4 that the *t*-distribution with an infinite number of degrees of freedom becomes identical with the normal distribution and the tables can thus be used to obtain critical values of the latter.

A word of warning. Be careful to avoid confusion because the tables given in this text give the critical values corresponding to various probability levels, whereas in some texts these are represented as percentages and as a consequence the tables are labelled, for example, as 'Percentage points' rather than 'Critical values of the *t*-distribution'. This simply means the *P* values 0.05, 0.025, etc. are labelled 5%, 2.5%, etc.

In the case of the normal distribution, a few of the values of Z which exclude some of the more common percentages in the right-hand 'tail' are as follows:

Probability	Percentage probability	Z
0.005	0.5	2.576
0.01	1.0	2.326
0.025	2.5	1.960
0.05	5.0	1.645

Example 5.3

This simple example illustrates the use of a table giving percentage points of a distribution. The cholesterol level in the blood was measured in a sample of ten patients who had suffered a heart attack and the mean was found to be 5.84 mmol/l. The level in a large number of individuals who had not suffered such an attack, for the purpose of this example taken to be the value for the population at large, was also measured and found to have a mean and standard deviation of 5.05 and 1.20 mmol/l respectively. As in the previous example, for simplicity, we make the assumption that the standard deviation of the latter measurement also applies to the sample.

The question that is asked is: is the blood cholesterol level in patients who have had a heart attack higher than in 'healthy' individuals?

The null and alternative hypotheses are:

$$H_0: \quad \mu = \mu_0$$

$$H_1: \quad \mu > \mu_0$$

and $n = 10$, $\bar{x} = 5.84$, $\mu_0 = 5.05$ and $\sigma = 1.20$, therefore:

$$Z = \frac{\bar{x} - \mu_0}{\sigma/\sqrt{n}}$$

$$= \frac{5.84 - 5.05}{1.20/\sqrt{10}}$$

$$= 2.08$$

Referring to the full normal distribution table (Table A), it can be seen that the probability that Z will be less than 2.08 (i.e. the CDF, the 'cumulative density function') is 0.9812, and therefore the probability that it will exceed 2.08 is $1 - 0.9812 = 0.0188$. Thus it can be said that $P = 0.0188$.

If, however, only a table of critical values of Z is available, or, alternatively, the t-distribution (Table B in Appendix VI) at an infinite number of degrees of freedom (where the normal and t-distributions become identical) may be used, we can see that the calculated value of Z, i.e. 2.08, lies between the values corresponding to a probability of 0.01 and 0.025, or 1% and 2.5%, so it would be reported that:

$$0.01 < P < 0.025$$

Clearly, at the 5% level of significance, H_0 would be rejected and it would be said that the difference is significant. Alternatively, since P is also less than 0.025 it might be said that 'the difference is significant at 2.5%', which means, of course, that the probability that the observed difference has occurred by random variation is less than 0.025, or 2.5%, and by implication greater than the next commonly quoted lower level. Thus the null hypothesis would be rejected in favour of the alternative and it would be concluded that the patients who have suffered a heart attack had a higher blood cholesterol level than the 'normal' subjects.

One- and two-way tests

Referring once again to Example 5.2, note that, because the normal distribution is symmetrical, there is a similar probability of 0.006 that a value of -3.24, or less, will occur by chance. In other words, the probability that a sample of 40 individuals would yield a mean which *differs* by 3.24 standard deviations from the population mean by random chance is $2 \times 0.0006 = 0.0012$. Thus, if the alternative, or experimental, hypothesis had simply been that the mean of the population from which the sample was taken was *not* 72, it would have been stated:

$$H_1: \ \mu \neq \mu_0$$

whereupon a 'two-way' or 'non-directional' test would be conducted, as opposed to the first alternative hypothesis considered above which constitutes a 'one-way' or 'directional' test. Thus, it is the nature of the experimental hypothesis which determines whether a one- or two-tailed test is performed, i.e. whether the critical values of Z occur in one, or both 'tails' of the normal distribution. Figure 4.10 shows the two tails for the critical values at $\alpha = 0.05$, where the area is 0.025 in each tail, and $Z = \pm 1.96$.

To summarize, in all cases:

$$H_0: \ \mu = \mu_0$$

For a one-way, or directional test two possibilities exist:

$$H_1: \ \mu > \mu_0$$

or

$$H_1: \ \mu < \mu_0$$

For a two-way, or non-directional test:

$$H_1: \ \mu \neq \mu_0$$

For a one-way test at the 5% level of significance, the critical value of Z is Z_α or $Z_{0.05}$ so that the null hypothesis is rejected when Z is greater than 1.645 if the alternative hypothesis is $H_1: \ \mu > \mu_0$, or when $Z < -1.645$ if $H_1: \ \mu < \mu_0$. For a two-way test, the critical values are $\pm Z_{\alpha/2}$ or $\pm Z_{0.025}$, i.e. $Z = 1.96$ so the null hypothesis is rejected if Z falls outside this range.

The normal distribution and the Z-test have been considered here as an introduction to significance testing and because this distribution is the most fundamental of all those which we shall encounter. It is, however, much more likely that, when comparing means, the standard deviation of the population will not be known and will be estimated from a small sample, or samples, in which case the t-distribution is used and a t-test is performed. Such a situation is considered in Chapter 6.

Summary

A RANDOM SAMPLE is one in which every member of the population has an equal chance of being included.

THE STANDARD ERROR OF THE MEAN. If many samples are taken from a given population, the means of those samples will follow a normal distribution with a mean equal to the population mean, and a standard deviation of these means is given by $\sigma/\sqrt{n}$. The latter is usually referred to as 'the standard error of the mean'.

THE STANDARD NORMAL DEVIATE (Z) represents the difference between any given value of the random variable (observation or measurement) and the mean in units of standard deviation of that random variable.

THE NULL HYPOTHESIS asserts, as the name suggests, that no difference exists between the quantities which are being compared. If sufficient evidence is found, this hypothesis is rejected in favour of the alternative or experimental hypothesis.

THE ALTERNATIVE OR EXPERIMENTAL HYPOTHESIS determines whether a one-way (directional) or two-way (non-directional) test is performed.

THE LEVEL OF SIGNIFICANCE at which we choose to work indicates the risk that we are prepared to take in wrongly rejecting the null hypothesis in favour of the alternative. For example, at the 5% level of significance, we reject H_0 if the probability that our observed result has occurred by chance is less than 5%. But, of course, there is a probability, though less than 0.05, or 5%, that it *has* occurred by chance. The level of significance is often given the symbol α.

THE P-VALUE is the probability that the observed effect has occurred by chance. When using statistical tables, this generally can only be quoted as a range rather than a specific value. The latter, however, can be obtained from many computer packages.

LEVEL OF CONFIDENCE is an indication of the confidence with which we may reject the null hypothesis. It is represented as a percentage and is given by $100(1-\alpha)\%$, where α is the significance level.

Exercises for Chapter 5

Exercise 5.1

Assume that the population mean systolic blood pressure of 20 to 25-year old males is 120 mmHg. A sample of 40 members of an athletic club within this age group were found to have a mean and standard deviation of 115.8 and 20 mmHg respectively.

(a) Calculate the standard error of the mean of a sample of size 40.
(b) Test the hypothesis that the club members have a significantly lower blood pressure than the population at large at the 5% level.
(c) What is the value of the mean blood pressure of the sample which would represent a significant difference at the 5% level?

Exercise 5.2

The overall mean and standard deviation mark in a certain examination was found to be 62.3 and 9.8, respectively. In a particular institution, a group of 39 students were found to have a mean of 65.6 in the same examination. Assume the standard deviation in the sample is unchanged. Is the mean of the sample significantly different from the overall (population) mean?

Exercise 5.3

The mean skinfold thickness of a large number of male subjects measured at the triceps mid-point has been estimated at 14.1 mm with a standard deviation of 5.2 mm.

(a) Estimate the standard error of the mean of a random sample of 12 male subjects.
(b) Put 90% confidence limits on an estimate of the mean of such a sample.
(c) Estimate the interquartile range of skinfold thickness of the population as a whole.

Exercise 5.4

The pinch grip strength (kg) at the tip of the thumb and forefinger of the dominant hand was measured on 30 male subjects within the age range 25–29 years. The following data were recorded:

7.0 4.7 7.7 7.2 7.0 7.5 8.1 8.1 7.8 7.4 6.0 7.5 9.4 7.0 7.6

6.5 6.6 8.5 6.4 8.5 6.6 8.2 8.5 4.8 8.6 8.2 7.7 8.4 7.0 7.2

(a) Put 95% confidence limits on an estimation of the population mean for this age group.
(b) The tip pinch grip strength was measured in a group of 325 males in the 60–69 age group and was found to have a mean of 6.69 with a standard deviation of 1.22 kg. What percentage of the population in this age group would be expected to have a tip pinch grip strength (i) greater than 7.0, (ii) less than 5.0, and (iii) between 6.0 and 8.0 kg.

Exercise 5.5

The mean hip flexion for 110 young adult subjects was found to be 125.2°. In the case of 22 of the subjects the measurement exceeded 140°. Estimate the standard deviation for this measurement.

6

Comparison of Means with the *t*-test

Contents
—The *t*-test: One sample.
            Two independent samples.
            Paired or related samples.
—Confidence intervals on estimations.

Introduction

If the standard deviation for a population is known, the normal distribution may be used to compare means. If however, as is usually the case, this is not known and is estimated from a small sample (generally taken to mean of size less than 30), the *t*-distribution, which is dependent on sample size, is used.

This distribution is similar to the normal distribution, but there is an additional variability as a result of the fact that the standard deviation is estimated from the sample, and will thus vary from one sample to another. In addition, this variability increases as the sample size decreases, so that the *t*-distribution is dependent on the size of the sample, or, more exactly, the number of *degrees of freedom*. You will recall from Chapter 2 that the number of degrees of freedom in a sample is $(n - 1)$ where n is the number of observations or measurements in that sample.

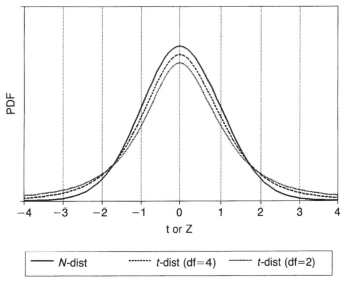

Figure 6.1 *Distribution curves showing the relationship between the normal and t-distributions*

Figure 6.1 shows the *t*-distribution for samples of two different sizes compared with the normal distribution.

You will recall, from Chapter 5, that when the number of degrees of freedom is very large, strictly infinite, the normal and *t*-distributions become identical.

Parametric and non-parametric tests

A *parametric test* is one in which one or more parameters, for example, the mean and standard deviation of the population from which the sample, or samples, have been taken are estimated, and the assumption is made that the population, at least approximately, follows a normal distribution.

Remember that the mean and standard deviation (or variance) of a sample are known as *statistics*, because they vary from one sample to another, whilst of a population they are known as *parameters* because they have fixed values, even if these are unknown. Also, a sample statistic is an estimation of the corresponding population parameter. Such tests, of which the t-test is one, should only be used with interval, or ratio, data.

A *non-parametric test*, or as it is sometimes called, a *distribution-free test*, makes no assumptions about the nature of the distribution, nor does it involve estimation of population parameters. Such tests are used when data is ranked and are considered in Chapter 9.

Parametric tests in general are said to be fairly 'robust', that is, they are not influenced to a great extent by deviations from normality, unless these are severe, and opinions differ regarding the importance of non-parametric tests. They are, however, in common use.

The t-test

The t-test, which is a parametric test, is sometimes referred to as the 'Student's t-test', not because it was designed for students, but because it was published by William Gossett under the pseudonym 'Student' in 1908. Gossett was at the time working for a well-known brewery in Ireland which did not permit its employees to publish research, so he resorted to the use of the pseudonym.

The definition of t is, in principle, the same as Z, i.e.

$$t = \frac{\text{(Random variable)} - \text{(Population parameter)}}{\text{SE (Random variable)}} \tag{6.1}$$

where SE (Random variable) is the 'standard error' or standard deviation of the random variable.

The definition, however, may take one of several forms depending on the nature of the random variable and the type of test employed.

In general, there are three types of t-test, namely:

—A one-sample t-test.
—An independent sample, or two-sample, t-test.
—A paired sample or related t-test.

These three types are now considered individually.

A one-sample *t*-test

This test compares the mean of a sample with a specified population mean when the standard deviation of the population is not known so must be estimated from the sample. This is, perhaps, the least common form of the *t*-test. Consider the following example as an illustration:

Example 6.1

Assume that, within a specified age range, the population as a whole has an average systolic blood pressure of 120.9 mmHg. The blood pressure of a group of eight individuals, comprising our statistical sample, who had been taking a diet considered to be unhealthy was also measured with the following results:

134   126   119   143   114   127   116   137

Test the hypothesis that the unhealthy diet causes an increase in blood pressure. Put into other words, the question that is being asked is: can it be concluded that this unhealthy diet leads to an increase in systolic blood pressure?

Using the statistics mode on a hand calculator, the mean and standard deviation will be found to be 127.0 and 10.42 mmHg respectively.

The principle of the test is identical with the test that we carried out in Chapter 3 to determine the significance of the correlation coefficient. The null hypothesis is straightforward, and, as always, it is that there is no difference between the two quantities being compared, in this case the mean of the population from which the sample was taken and the specified population mean.

The experimental or alternative hypothesis is that the unhealthy diet increases the blood pressure, so we perform a one-way test. This seems to be reasonable in the circumstances, because, if the diet affected the blood pressure, we would expect it to cause an increase rather than a decrease. Thus a directional or one-way test is employed, so that the following hypotheses would be tested:

$$H_0: \ \mu = \mu_0 \qquad H_0: \ \mu = 120.9$$
$$\text{or}$$
$$H_1: \ \mu > \mu_0 \qquad H_1: \ \mu > 120.9$$

where μ_0 represents the specified population mean, in this case 120.9, μ is the mean of the population from which the sample was taken, $\bar{x}$ is the mean of the sample and is an estimate of μ. The standard deviation, s, measured from the sample, is an estimate of the standard deviation of that population, and it is because the standard deviation of the population is not known that we use a t-test rather than a Z-test.

For a one-sample test t takes the form:

$$t_0 = \frac{(\bar{x} - \mu_0)}{s/\sqrt{n}} \tag{6.2}$$

because the sample statistic is the mean of the sample of size 8, and the standard error of the sample statistic is $s/\sqrt{n}$.

Substituting in the above equation (6.2) enables t to be evaluated:

$$t_0(\text{df} = 7) = \frac{(127.0 - 120.9)}{10.42/\sqrt{8}}$$

$$= 1.66$$

The subscript '0' is often used to indicate the 'observed' value of t, and also there are 8 observations, or measurements, thus 7 degrees of freedom (df). From the tables for the t-distribution (Table B) we find that, at 7 degrees of freedom, for a one-way test:

$$t_{0.10} = 1.415$$

$$t_{0.05} = 1.895$$

i.e. by chance alone, t may take values as large as, or larger than, 1.415 or 1.895 with probabilities 0.10 and 0.05, respectively. The observed value, 1.66, for a one-way test, lies between the two, and thus has a probability of between 0.05 and 0.10 of having occurred by chance. Therefore we conclude:

$$0.05 < P < 0.10$$

So that, if we are working at the 5% level of significance, there is insufficient evidence to reject the null hypothesis in favour of the alternative, so we conclude that the diet does not increase the blood pressure. This is because there is a greater than 5% probability that the observed difference between the sample mean (127.0) and the specified population mean (120.9) has occurred by chance.

Summary of the rationale for the *t*-test

Using the *t*-distribution we calculate the probability that a sample of size 8 (7 degrees of freedom) would have a mean of 127.0 or more as a result of random variation if it is taken from a population with mean 120.9 and if the standard deviation of the sample is 10.42.

If this probability is greater than our chosen level of significance, in this case, 0.05 or 5%, we conclude that this is a relatively likely event and therefore infer that the difference *is* the result of random variable, i.e. the null hypothesis is accepted.

If the probability is less than 5%, we conclude that it is too unlikely an event to occur by chance if the mean of the population from which the sample was taken is the same as the specified population mean, i.e. the null hypothesis is rejected in favour of the alternative, or experimental hypothesis.

The *P*-value represents the probability that the observed result would occur by chance if the null hypothesis is true.

Remember that, if we choose to work at the 5% level of significance, we are saying that we are prepared to accept a 5% chance of being wrong if we reject the null hypothesis, because, for a sample of size 8, there is a 5% probability that the value of *t* will exceed 1.895 by chance if the null hypothesis is true. Thus, if our observed value of *t* is greater than 1.895, we would reject the null hypothesis even though there is a 5% probability that *t* will exceed this value by random variation.

Remember also, as was pointed out in Chapter 3, it is better to quote a *P*-value, or at least a range of values obtained from the tables, rather than to simply say the null hypothesis is rejected at the 5% level of significance.

The chosen level of significance

Experience suggests that, for most purposes, 5% is about the best value to use. If you have forgotten the arguments relating to this choice, refer to Chapter 5 and the comments following the Z-test.

The following example illustrates a circumstance where a lower level of significance may be appropriate.

Example 6.2

Imagine that it has been suggested that a new treatment for a particular injury is more effective and will bring about a cure much more quickly. You wish to introduce this new treatment, but it requires the purchase of some expensive equipment. The finance committee needs to be convinced. The average number of treatments required using the existing method is known to be eight.

The new equipment is acquired on loan and used to treat a sample of ten patients. The number of treatments required for each patient was as follows:

$$6 \quad 9 \quad 5 \quad 9 \quad 7 \quad 7 \quad 5 \quad 7 \quad 4 \quad 8$$

Calculate t and test at the 5% and 1% levels of significance.

In this case, we conduct a one-way test because the experimental hypothesis is that the new method results in a decrease, rather than just a change, in the average number of treatments necessary to effect a recovery.

From the data t may be calculated:

$$t_0(\text{df} = 9) = \frac{\bar{x} - \mu_0}{s/\sqrt{n}}$$

$$= \frac{6.7 - 8}{1.703/\sqrt{10}}$$

$$= -2.414$$

The fact that our observed value is negative (-2.414) simply means that the sample mean is less than the specified population mean by

2.414 standard errors of the mean. As far as the interpretation is concerned, this does not present a problem because, as with the normal distribution, the *t*-distribution is symmetrical, so that the probability that *t* will exceed 2.414 by chance is exactly the same as the probability that it will be less than −2.414.

The 'critical value' of *t* with 9 degrees of freedom at the 5% level of significance is found from Table B to be 1.833 for a one-way test. Thus, since the calculated value of *t* is numerically greater than 1.833, there is a less than 5% probability that the observed value of *t*, and hence the observed sample mean, has occurred by chance. Thus, at this level of significance, you would reject the null hypothesis in favour of the alternative and conclude that the new method does reduce the number of necessary treatments.

This result may well be presented to the finance committee as evidence that the new method is more effective than the old.

Remember that, when working at the 5% level of significance you are accepting a 5% chance of rejecting the null hypothesis when it is true. The committee, however, may well respond by saying that they are not prepared to take a 5% chance of being wrong because a change would incur a considerable capital outlay, but they are prepared to accept a 1% chance of being wrong.

The calculated value of *t*, of course, still stands, but we must refer again to Table B where we find that the observed value (2.414) falls between the critical values of *t* at 2.5% and 1%, i.e. there is a greater than 1% chance that this value of *t* has occurred by chance so that, if the null hypothesis is rejected, the probability that this is wrong is greater than 1%. So, sadly, the finance committee will not permit you to introduce the new method of treatment.

The final conclusion, as before, is given as:

$$0.01 < P < 0.025$$

Many computer packages, such as MINITAB, will give a specific value for the probability, or *P*-value, for a given experimental value of *t*. That is the probability that this value, or larger, would occur by chance if the null hypothesis is actually true. Using MINITAB we find:

$$P = 0.0195$$

which, of course, lies between 0.01 and 0.025.

Level of confidence

As with the Z-test, or any other test of significance, if the null hypothesis is rejected at, say, the 5% level, we are saying that there is a 5% chance that we are mistaken, but a 95% chance that we are not. Thus alternative ways of stating the conclusion are:

(a)   the difference is significant at the 5% level; or
(b)   the null hypothesis may be rejected with 95% confidence.

An independent sample t-test

This test is used to compare two samples when each sample contains data obtained independently of each other. For example, if it is required to compare the blood pressure of two groups of people, such as males and females.

Example 6.3

An experiment was conducted to see if a significant difference existed in blood pressure between male and female subjects. For this purpose, two samples, which were matched as far as possible with regard to age and lifestyles, were selected. They comprised eight males and ten females respectively.

The blood pressure (mmHg) of each subject was measured with the following results:

Males   126 106 127 121 126 129 134 126

Females 130 133 132 131 124 137 120 148 123 128

Using a hand calculator it is found that:

$$\bar{x}_M = 124.38 \quad s_M = 8.262$$
$$\bar{x}_F = 130.60 \quad s_F = 7.975$$

In this case the 'random variable' is the difference between the two sample means:

$$(\bar{x}_M - \bar{x}_F) \quad \text{or} \quad (\bar{x}_F - \bar{x}_M)$$

The population parameter with which we are comparing it is zero. This is because the null hypothesis states that there is no difference between the means of the populations from which the samples were taken, i.e. the difference between them is zero. We then take the observed difference and, in the light of the calculated standard deviations, consider the probability, by calculating the *t*-statistic, that this difference might occur by chance alone.

It can be shown that the standard error of the difference is given by:

$$s_P\sqrt{\frac{1}{n_M} + \frac{1}{n_F}} \tag{6.3}$$

where s_p is the *pooled estimate of the standard deviation*:

$$s_p = \sqrt{\frac{(n_M - 1)s_M^2 + (n_F - 1)s_F^2}{(n_M - 1) + (n_F - 1)}}$$

$$= \sqrt{\frac{7(8.262)^2 + 9(7.975)^2}{7 + 9}}$$

$$= 8.102$$

We can see that this is simply the square root of the average variance, where the latter has been 'weighted' according to the size (number of degrees of freedom) of each sample, thus each sample contributes to the variance estimate of the population according to its size. It is reasonable to accept that the larger sample will contribute more to this estimate than the smaller sample.

The assumption is made in this case that the two variances (or standard deviations) are not significantly different and both are estimates of a common population value. Strictly a non-directional *F*-test (see Chapter 8) should be conducted to verify this.

Note that the total number of degrees of freedom is the sum of the number for each sample.

Thus the *t* statistic becomes:

$$t = \frac{(\bar{x}_F - \bar{x}_M) - (\mu_F - \mu_M)}{s_P\sqrt{\dfrac{1}{n_M} + \dfrac{1}{n_F}}} \qquad (6.5)$$

$$t_0(\mathrm{df} = 16) = \frac{(130.60 - 124.38) - 0}{8.102\sqrt{\dfrac{1}{8} + \dfrac{1}{10}}}$$

$$= 1.62$$

It is quite arbitrary whether the difference in the sample means is taken as $(\bar{x}_F - \bar{x}_M)$ or $(\bar{x}_M - \bar{x}_F)$ so it is convenient to take the positive option and thereby reduce the risk of confusion. A two-way test is appropriate because the experimental hypothesis is that the means of the samples are *different* from each other. Thus the relevant hypotheses are:

$$\begin{array}{ccc} H_0: \ \mu_F = \mu_M & & H_0: \ \mu_F - \mu_M = 0 \\ & \text{or} & \\ H_1: \ \mu_F \neq \mu_M & & H_1: \ \mu_F - \mu_M \neq 0 \end{array}$$

Reference to the table for the critical values of the t-distribution (Table B) for a two-way test at 16 degrees of freedom, i.e. $(n_F - 1) + (n_M - 1)$, shows that:

$$t_{0.20} = 1.337$$

$$t_{0.10} = 1.746$$

The observed value of t is 1.62, i.e. the observed difference between the means of the samples is 1.62 standard deviations (standard errors of the difference between the means) from zero. The tables indicate that the probability that this should occur by chance is between 0.1 and 0.2, or between 10% and 20%, i.e.

$$0.10 < P < 0.20$$

Thus, there is insufficient evidence to reject the null hypothesis. We would therefore conclude that there is not a significant difference between the blood pressure of males and females.

Remember that the significance level for a given value of t for a two-way test is double that for a one-way test because we consider the probability that an observed value of the test statistic will differ, in either direction, in this case by 1.62 standard deviations.

Also, the larger the observed value of t, the less likely it is that it has occurred by chance, thus the observed value of 1.62, being smaller than the critical positive value at 10% (for a two-way test), means that the probability that the observed value occurred by chance is greater than 10%.

A *t*-test for significantly different variances

If it transpires that, as a result of conducting an F-test (see Chapter 8) it is concluded that the variances of the two samples *are* significantly different, then the value of t and the number of degrees of freedom (rounded to the nearest whole number) are calculated rather differently, using the following equations:

$$t_0 = \frac{(\bar{x}_A - \bar{x}_B) = (\mu_A - \mu_B)}{\sqrt{\dfrac{s_A^2}{n_A} + \dfrac{s_B^2}{n_B}}} \qquad \text{df} = \frac{(s_A^2/n_A + s_B^2 n_B)}{\dfrac{(s_A^2/n_A)^2}{n_A - 1} + \dfrac{(s_B^2/n_B)^2}{(n_B - 1)}}$$

$$(6.6)$$

If a pooled t-test is used when it is not appropriate, that is, when the two sample standard deviations *are* significantly different, the calculated value of t may indicate a higher significance than actually exists. The difference, however, unless the standard deviations and/or sample sizes are very dissimilar, is often fairly small.

Paired or related sample *t*-test

The crucial point about this test is that each observation has an identifiable partner. In Example 6.2, the blood pressure was measured on different individuals and each observation was independent of any other. If, however, measurement was made on each subject under two different conditions, we have a pair of observations which are compared with each other. An inter-method reliability test is an example of such a comparison.

Example 6.4

The blood pressure of six subjects was measured using both a manual and an automatic method to see whether the results are comparable.

	Manual method (M)	Automatic method (A)	Difference (M − A)
Mr Smith	125	125	0
Mrs Jones	122	118	4
Mr Peters	134	132	2
Miss Johnson	118	119	−1
Mr Scott	132	129	3
Mrs Franks	129	127	2

This test differs from the independent sample t-test considered above because we are concerned here with the difference, if any, between the measurements using each method. We are not concerned with variability between the subjects. It is clear that there would be no point comparing the result of a manual measurement on Mr Smith with the automatic measurement on Mrs Jones. The 'random variable' is now the difference between each pair of measurements, and we consider the question: is the average difference between each pair of measurements significantly different from zero? Thus the relevant hypotheses for a two-way test are:

$$H_0: \quad \mu_d = \text{zero}$$

$$H_1: \quad \mu_d \neq \text{zero}$$

The t-statistic now becomes:

$$t_0 = \frac{\bar{d} - \mu_d}{s_d / \sqrt{n}} \qquad (6.7)$$

where:

$s_d =$ the standard deviation of the differences—obtained with a calculator.

$n =$ the number of differences, i.e. the number of pairs of measurements. Thus $s_d / \sqrt{n}$ becomes the 'standard error' of the mean of the differences.

μ_d = the population value for the difference with which we are comparing the observed average difference. If there is no difference between the manual and automatic method of measurement, this will be zero, i.e. the null hypothesis is H_0: μ_d = zero.

$\bar{d}$ = the average difference. Note that when calculating this mean and s_d, the values for the differences, including the sign and any zero values, must be entered into the calculator.

From the data:

$$\bar{d} = 1.667 \quad s_d = 1.862 \quad n = 6$$

As before, it is quite arbitrary whether the difference is measured as $(M - A)$ or $(A - M)$ so, for convenience, we take the former to obtain a positive value for t.

So t may now be calculated:

$$t_0(df = 5) = \frac{1.667}{1.862/\sqrt{6}}$$

$$= 2.193$$

From Table B in Appendix VI, we find that the appropriate critical values of t for a two-way test at 5 degrees of freedom are:

$$t_{0.10} = \pm 2.015$$

$$t_{0.05} = +2.571$$

Remember, this means that for a two-way test, if the null hypothesis is true, there is a 5% chance that it will fall outside the range ± 2.571 and a 10% chance that it will fall outside the range ± 2.015. The observed value, 2.193, lies between these two so that we would report that:

$$0.05 < P < 0.10$$

So, at the 5% level of significance, we would accept the null hypothesis and conclude that the two methods yield results which are not significantly different from each other.

If, however, experience had led us to suspect that the automatic method yields a lower result than the manual method, a one-way test would have been appropriate and the relevant hypotheses would have been:

$$H_0: \mu_d = \text{zero}$$

$$H_1: \mu_d > \text{zero}$$

whereupon:

$$0.025 < P < 0.05$$

so that the null hypothesis would now be rejected in favour of the alternative at the 5% level of significance.

It is worth reiterating here that if we choose a 5% level of significance for our test, we are prepared to accept a 5% chance of being wrong if we reject the null hypothesis. This is because, of course, there is a 5% chance that t will be greater than the critical value, in this case 2.015 (for a one-way test), even if the null hypothesis *is* true.

In the case of a two-way, or non-directional test, the 5% probability is split, so that there is a 2.5% probability that t will be greater than $+2.571$, and a 2.5% probability that it will be less than -2.571 by chance alone, giving a total of 5%. Thus if the numerical value of t is greater than 2.571, whether it is positive or negative, we would reject the null hypothesis in favour of the alternative, or experimental, hypothesis with a 5% chance of being wrong, or with 95% confidence that we are right.

The rationale for a paired sample or related t-test

When considering repeated measurements on a number of different subjects, why are we not able to perform a normal t-test on the means of each group? The reason for this is best explained by looking at a simple example:

Consider the following 'before' and 'after' measurements on six subjects:

Subject	Before (B)	After (A)	A − B
A	12	14	2
B	13	14	1
C	11	13	2
D	12	13	1
E	13	14	1
F	13	13	0

A paired sample *t*-test (see Example 6.4) yields: $t_0(df = 5) = 3.80$. From the tables we conclude that for a two-way test, $0.01 < P < 0.02$, i.e. the difference is significant.

An independent sample *t*-test comparing the means of the two groups 'before' and 'after' yields: $t_0(df = 10) = 2.91$, for which the P value lies within the same range. Thus, in this case, we would draw the same conclusion whichever test we had used. But, if we change the data by alternately adding and subtracting 5 from each pair of values:

Subject	Before (B)	After (A)	A − B
A	17	19	2
B	8	9	1
C	16	18	2
D	7	8	1
E	18	19	1
F	8	8	0

The column containing the differences remains the same, so the result of a paired sample test, of course, is exactly as above.

The mean of each column also remains the same ($\bar{x}_B = 12.33$, $\bar{x}_A = 13.5$), however, the independent sample *t*-test now yields $t_U(df − 10) − 0.37$, which we can see from Table B shows that $P > 40\%$. Reference to the computer package MINITAB tells us that, actually, $P = 0.72$ or 72%. Thus, there is a 72% probability that the observed differences in the means of the two groups has occurred by chance. This is because the variability between the different subjects within each group has now become very large so that the difference between the means is much more likely to be a matter of chance. In the first example, this was very small and therefore the differences between the means was significant. This 'within group' (between subject) variability is eliminated in the paired sample test.

Confidence intervals when estimating a mean

Let us assume that it is required to estimate the average time taken to cure a particular muscular injury using a certain technique. This may be achieved by collecting data from a number of patients suffering from this injury and determining the mean in the usual way. Two sets of data, however, may have the same mean but have considerably different variabilities. An estimate of the population mean may be given together with a 'confidence interval', of which the minimum and maximum values are known as the 'confidence limits' which depend upon the variability or the standard error of the mean. The smaller the standard error of the mean, the narrower is the confidence interval and the more accurate is the estimate of the population mean.

Consider the following example:

Example 6.5

The following data represent the number of therapy sessions required to achieve a cure for six patients.

$$12 \quad 13 \quad 12 \quad 14 \quad 16 \quad 17$$

The mean of this sample is an estimate of the 'population mean', that is the average number of sessions that we would calculate if we were able to consider every single person suffering from this particular condition. In addition, we can indicate the reliability of this estimate by quoting the 95% confidence interval.

The mean and standard deviation for this sample may readily be obtained using a hand calculator and will be found to be 14.00 and 2.10 respectively. Quoting the standard deviation does, of course give an indication of the variability, although it is, perhaps, more satisfactory to quote a confidence interval, e.g. at 95%.

Referring to Equation 6.2 we see that t may be represented:

$$t = \frac{\bar{x} - \mu}{s / \sqrt{n}}$$

where the value of t is chosen to reflect the confidence interval required. Thus, for a 95% confidence interval we require the two values of t which will include a probability of 0.95, that is the two values which will show a probability of 0.025 in each tail of the distribution, which, because of its symmetry are numerically identical, differing only in sign. From Table B we find this critical value of t with 5 degrees of freedom is ±2.571. This is because there is a probability of 0.025 that the difference between the sample and population means will be plus or minus this number of standard errors of the mean.

Thus, Equation 6.7 may be rearranged to give:

$$\mu = \bar{x} \pm t_{0.025}(s/\sqrt{n}) \tag{6.8}$$

i.e. at 5 degrees of freedom:

$$\mu = \bar{x} \pm 2.571(2.10/\sqrt{6})$$
$$= 14.00 \pm 2.20$$

i.e. $11.8 < \mu < 16.2$

Thus we have 95% confidence that the population mean lies within this range. Note that this is not the same as saying that the population mean has a 95% probability of falling within this range, because, of course, it is a 'parameter' and therefore has a fixed value. What we are saying is that we have 95% confidence that we have identified a range within which it will be included.

In contrast, assume the data had been as follows:

21   17   11   12   10   13

The mean is exactly the same as above, namely 14.00, but the data are more variable with a standard deviation of 4.20. The 95% confidence interval in this case is calculated in the same way, and it can be seen that the interval is considerably wider, i.e.

$$\mu = \bar{x} \pm 2.571(4.20/\sqrt{6})$$
$$= 14.00 \pm 4.41$$

i.e. $9.6 < \mu < 18.4$

So that, in the first case, we have a 95% confidence that the true mean lies within the range 11.8 to 16.2, and in the second case, because of the greater variability, the range is extended, namely 9.6 to 18.4.

Summary

A ONE-SAMPLE t-TEST compares the mean of the population from which a sample has been taken with a specified population mean.

A TWO-SAMPLE OR INDEPENDENT SAMPLE t-TEST compares the means of the populations from which two independent samples have been taken, e.g. measurements on different subjects.

THE NUMBER OF DEGREES OF FREEDOM for a two-sample test is dependent upon whether the two variances are significantly different.

A PAIRED-SAMPLE OR RELATED t-TEST is conducted when repeated measures are involved on a number of different subjects, e.g. 'before' and 'after' measurements on each subject. The crucial point of recognition is that each observation must have an identifiable partner.

CONFIDENCE LIMITS on the estimated population mean may be determined from the sample mean and standard deviation, together with the appropriate values of t.

Exercises for Chapter 6

Exercise 6.1

A study was undertaken to determine whether relaxation training with biofeedback is able to reduce hypertension. Two groups of hypertensive subjects, A and B, were randomly assigned to receive training (ten subjects) and to act as a control (eight subjects). The following data show the reduction in systolic blood pressure (mmHg) after eight weeks:

Training (A):   22   17   27   9   25   0   −8   27   13   4

Control (B):   −4   −7   −8   8   −1   0   10   7

The negative values, of course, indicate an increase in the blood pressure.

(a) Do you think the training was successful at the 5% level of significance?
(b) What are the 98% confidence limits on the reduction of blood pressure in each group?
(c) Put 95% confidence limits on the difference between the mean reduction of blood pressure in each group.

Exercise 6.2

A comparison was made of the peak expiratory flow (PEF) of a group A of six asthmatic young adults with a group B of eight without respiratory problems. The following data were collected:

| Group A | 591 484 509 524 493 508 534 566 |
| Group B | 483 413 518 478 470 474 |

Is there a significant difference between the groups at the 5% level?

Exercise 6.3

An experiment was conducted to test the effect of a measured dose of whisky on reaction time. Eight volunteers had reaction time measured before, and ten minutes after, consumption:

		Mr A	Mr B	Mr C	Mr D	Mr E	Mr F	Mr G	Mr H
Reaction times	Before	0.11	0.14	0.20	0.20	0.22	0.21	0.21	0.23
	After	0.14	0.17	0.19	0.21	0.22	0.24	0.25	0.25

Can it be concluded that the alcohol increases the reaction time?

Exercise 6.4

The systolic blood pressure of a group of ten apparently healthy males in the age group 45 to 54 was measured before and after a standard exercise:

Subject:

A	B	C	D	E	F	G	H	I	J

Before exercise BP/mmHg:

131	142	141	136	145	148	147	153	164	138

After exercise BP/mmHg:

141	145	139	146	153	155	150	153	163	140

(a) Is there a significant increase in the blood pressure after exercise at the 5% level?

(b) Put 95% confidence limits on the estimation of the mean increase in blood pressure.

Exercise 6.5

A class of 40 students was divided at random into two equal groups. Each group followed an introductory course in statistics. Group A was taught by conventional methods and Group B using a computer-based self-instruction scheme. The following marks were obtained:

Group A
60 51 56 56 58 54 59 53 54 65 55 51 45 60 55 59 69 58 64 48

Group B
59 56 55 60 56 48 53 54 52 59 55 62 71 64 68 66 56 56 64 70

(a) Determine the mean and standard deviation of each group.

(b) It has been claimed that the computer-based self-learning package is more effective. Can this claim be justified at the 5% level of significance?

(c) Put 95% confidence limits on the estimate of the mean for each group.

7

Comparing Proportions and Testing for Independence

Contents
—The chi-square test for independence.
—The chi-square distribution.
—Contingency tables.
—Tests with low expected frequencies.

Introduction

The chi-square distribution is used to test proportions when considering *nominal* or *categorical data*, which in general means that we have data which arise from counting people or events, whereupon they are put into categories. We can then compare the frequencies with which individuals or events occur, or the proportions, in each category under different conditions. The chi-square test is often called either a 'test for independence', or a 'goodness-of-fit test'.

A test for independence

If a questionnaire was given to a group of patients in a hospital, some male and some female, and they were asked to rate the treatment in a particular clinic as either 'poor', 'average' or 'good', the proportions in each of these categories for the males may then be compared with that for the females using a chi-square test (see later in this chapter). If the proportions are not significantly different it may be said that the answers to the questions are independent of the sex of the respondent, i.e. it is a test for independence.

The chi-square (χ^2) statistic is defined as follows:

$$\chi^2 = \sum \frac{(O - E)^2}{E} \qquad (7.1)$$

where χ is the Greek letter 'chi' (pronounced 'ki'), O is the 'observed value' and E is the 'expected value'. It is called chi-square to emphasize the fact that it cannot take negative values. Remember that $\sum$ means 'the sum of'.

In order to calculate a value for chi-square for a set of data, it is clearly necessary to obtain 'expected' values. It is sometimes possible to know these exactly, and at other times they must be determined from the data. A simple example will, perhaps, demonstrate the general nature of the chi-square test. This example has been chosen to illustrate this test because it is very simple to determine the expected values.

Example 7.1

Assume that we have a die and wish to determine whether it is true or loaded. We ask the question: when rolled, does each face of the cube have an equal chance of showing its number, i.e. is the probability of obtaining a 'one', the same as that for a 'two' or 'three' . . . or 'six'? If the die is rolled 120 times, the expected numbers may easily be calculated. There are six faces on the cube so we would 'expect' each face to appear in 1/6 of the total number of rolls, i.e. in 120 rolls we would expect 20 of each number to be obtained, although, in practice, of course, random effects will result in variation from this number.

Assume that in this experiment of 120 rolls of the die 15 'ones', 20 'twos', 24 'threes', 12 'fours', 22 'fives' and 27 'sixes' were obtained. The result, together with the 'expected' values given in brackets, employing the usual convention, may be set out as follows:

Score	One	Two	Three	Four	Five	Six
Frequency	15 (20)	20 (20)	24 (20)	12 (20)	22 (20)	27 (20)

Chi-square may now be calculated:

$$\chi_0^2(df = 5) = \frac{(15 - 20)^2}{20} + \frac{(20 - 20)^2}{20} + \frac{(24 - 20)^2}{20}$$
$$+ \frac{(12 - 20)^2}{20} + \frac{(22 - 20)^2}{20} + \frac{(27 - 20)^2}{20}$$
$$= 1.250 + 0.000 + 0.800$$
$$+ 3.200 + 0.200 + 2.450$$
$$= 7.90$$

Notes:

—The subscript 'o' indicates the 'observed' or calculated value of chi-square.

—There are six observed frequencies, so there are five degrees of freedom. In a chi-square test the number of degrees of freedom is given by the least number of expected values that must be specified, or calculated, in order to fix them all. In this case, if five of the expected values are fixed at 20, the sixth can only take the value of 20 if the total is 120.

It is clear from the definition that the minimum value for χ^2 is zero, which would be the case, of course, if all the observed values were equal to the expected values. The maximum value, in this case, 600, would be obtained if, for example, 120 sixes were thrown, although this value will always depend upon the particular set of data. If the die had been rolled, say, 60 times, the maximum would be 300, whereas the minimum remains at zero.

The appropriate hypotheses are:

$$H_0: p_1 = p_2 = p_3 = p_4 = p_5 = p_6$$
$$H_1: \text{not all proportions are equal}$$

where $p_1 = $ the proportion of throws resulting in a 'one', etc.

The question we are asking is: how large may χ^2 become before we consider it to be too large to have occurred by random variation when its 'true' value is zero, i.e. if the null hypothesis is true?

Reference to the table of critical values of χ^2 (Table C in Appendix VI) reveals that for five degrees of freedom:

$$\chi^2_{0.05} = 11.07 \qquad \chi^2_{0.10} = 9.24$$
$$\chi^2_{0.20} = 7.29 \qquad \chi^2_{0.30} = 6.06$$

That is, the probability that χ^2 will be as large as, or larger than 11.07 is 0.05, or 5%, larger than 9.24 is 10% and so on. The observed value of χ^2 was found to be 7.90, which lies between the values at 10% and 20%. Thus it would be said that:

$$0.10 < P < 0.20$$

This means there is a probability of between 10% and 20% that the observed value (7.90) has occurred by chance if the null hypothesis is true, i.e. there is no real difference between the proportions of each number obtained in the experiment.

If we choose to work at the 5% level of significance, which is the most usual, the null hypothesis must be accepted, so that we would conclude that there is no difference between the proportions in each category, i.e. the die was not loaded and that there is an equal probability of obtaining each score.

Remember that working at the 5% level of significance means that we reject the null hypothesis if the probability that the observed value of chi-square has occurred by chance is less than 5%, which is not so in this case.

Note that, as with other test statistics, the larger the observed value of chi-square, the less likely it is that the null hypothesis is true.

The chi-square distribution

It is, perhaps, worth spending a little time looking at the general nature of the chi-square distribution. It can be seen in Figure 7.1 that it is asymmetrical, and it is said to be 'skewed to the right'. Like the t-distribution, it also is dependent on the number of degrees of freedom, although the general shape is as shown in the figure,

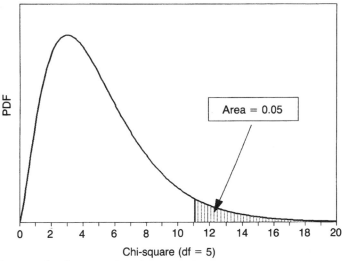

Figure 7.1 *The chi-square distribution with 5 degrees of freedom showing the probability that $\chi^2 > 11.07$*

provided there are at least three degrees of freedom. For fewer than three, the maximum PDF (probability density function) occurs at the origin where chi-square is equal to zero. Figure 7.1 shows the distribution with five degrees of freedom, and the shaded portion, when chi-square is greater than 11.07, contains 5% probability in the tail, i.e. when considering Example 7.1 above, if the null hypothesis is true, there is only a 5% chance that a value for chi-square above 11.07 will be observed. Thus, if our observed value had been 11.07 or larger, we would have rejected the null hypothesis and concluded that the probability of obtaining each number when rolling the die was not equal. But, of course, that means there is a probability of 5% (or less if χ^2 is greater than 11.07) that this value *has* occurred by chance, so there is a 5% chance that we would have been wrong in rejecting H_0.

The continuous χ^2 distribution has been calculated mathematically, but one can imagine how it could be obtained experimentally, although it would be a very time-consuming and tedious business and is not recommended. The above example would yield a suitable experiment for this purpose because the expected values are known exactly, and if the experiment, i.e. rolling the die 120 times, is repeated an extremely large number of

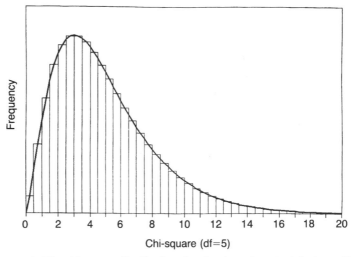

Figure 7.2 *The chi-square distribution showing how, in principle, it could be obtained by collecting data and preparing a histogram*

times and the value of chi-square is calculated in each case, a histogram may be constructed, with, say, a class width of 0.5, whereupon the shape would be similar to the continuous curve, becoming closer to it the larger the number of classes, and the narrower the class width, and the greater the quantity of data collected (see Figure 7.2). The vertical axis in that case would be the frequency of occurrence in each class.

Contingency tables

In the case of Example 7.1, the expected values are known exactly, which is fairly rare; it is much more common that these would be calculated from the collected data in the form of a 'contingency table', as illustrated in the following example.

Example 7.2

Consider again the example suggested at the beginning of this chapter and assume that a group of 120 patients, 70 male and 50 female were asked to rate the treatment they had received as 'poor', 'average' or 'good'.

Is there a significant difference between the response of the male and female patients? This question may be worded rather differently, namely: is the response to the questionnaire independent of the sex of the respondent?

The responses may be represented in a 'contingency table' as follows:

	Male	Female	Total
Poor	10 (8.167)	4 (5.833)	14
Average	26 (32.667)	30 (23.333)	56
Good	34 (29.167)	16 (20.833)	50
Total	70	50	120

The expected values are given in brackets. These are calculated by converting the totals in each column into the same ratio as the grand totals given in the right-hand column, for example, the 70 male respondents are divided into the ratio $14 : 56 : 50$. Thus the expected value in the male 'poor' cell is given by $(14/120) \times 70 = 8.167$, and in the male 'average' cell, by $(56/120) \times 70 = 32.667$, etc.

We should note that the sum of the expected values must, of course, add up to the total in the column. It is useful to check that this is so before continuing.

Chi-square may now be calculated:

$$\chi_0^2(\text{df} = 2) = \frac{(10 - 8.167)^2}{8.167} + \frac{(4 - 5.833)^2}{5.833} + \frac{(26 - 32.667)^2}{32.667}$$

$$+ \frac{(30 - 23.333)^2}{23.333} + \frac{(34 - 29.167)^2}{29.167}$$

$$+ \frac{(16 - 20.833)^2}{20.833}$$

$$= 0.411 + 0.576 + 1.361$$

$$+ 1.905 + 0.801 + 1.121$$

$$= 6.18$$

Care should be taken not to 'round off' the expected values too much because the square of a difference is being calculated and therefore small errors will be magnified.

The number of degrees of freedom is given by the least number of expected values that must be calculated in order to complete the table. There are two degrees of freedom in this example because it is necessary to calculate only two expected values, for example, if the values in the male 'poor' and 'average' cells are calculated, all the others may be obtained by subtraction from the totals. Alternatively, the number of degrees of freedom is given by $(c - 1)(r - 1)$, where c and r represent the number of columns and rows respectively.

Cells with low expected frequency

Opinions are divided with regard to the calculation of chi-square when the expected values are rather small, although the most commonly accepted practice is to ensure that no cells have an expected value less than unity, and no more than 20% have expected frequencies less than five. In the case of a 2×2 contingency table, the frequencies in the table should not total less than 20 and no cells should have an expected frequency less than 5.

If such circumstances do arise, the only alternatives, if the chi-square test is to be used, is either to collect more data, or to combine two or more of the groups. This is illustrated in the following example.

Example 7.3

A survey was conducted to determine whether smoking habits are independent of age and the following data were collected where the number of cigarettes smoked per day is tabulated against an age group.

Age range

Smoked/day	<24	25–44	45–64	>64
None	7	7	14	1
11–20	3	12	4	4
21–30	9	5	5	3
>30	4	3	5	5

The contingency table, together with the expected frequencies may be set up as follows:

Age range

Smoked /day	<24	25–44	45–64	>64	Total
None	7 (7.330)	7 (8.604)	14 (8.923)	1 (4.143)	29
11–20	3 (5.813)	12 (6.824)	4 (7.077)	4 (3.286)	23
21–30	9 (5.560)	5 (6.527)	5 (6.769)	3 (3.143)	22
>30	4 (4.297)	3 (5.044)	5 (5.231)	5 (2.429)	17
Total	23	27	28	13	91

The expected values, calculated as in Example 7.2, are given in brackets. Note that five of the 12 cells, i.e. 42%, have expected values less than 5. As mentioned above, a valid chi-square test can only be conducted if no more than 20% of the cells have expected values less than 5, so in this case an adjustment must be made. The problem arises because the age range >64 contains only 13 individuals—either some more data must be collected, or the two groups 45–64 and >64 may be combined, whereupon the contingency table becomes:

	<24	25–44	>44	Total
None	7 (7.330)	7 (8.604)	15 (13.066)	29
11–20	3 (5.813)	12 (6.824)	8 (10.363)	23
21–30	9 (5.560)	5 (6.527)	8 (9.912)	22
>30	4 (4.297)	3 (5.044)	10 (7.659)	17
Total	23	27	41	91

Now only a single cell has an expected value of less than 5 so that a valid chi-square test may be performed. This does mean, of course, that the conclusion is rather more limited.

The relevant hypotheses are:

$$H_0 : p_1 = p_2 = p_3$$

$$H_1 : \text{Not all proportions are equal}$$

and

$$\chi_0^2 = \frac{(7 - 7.330)^2}{7.330} + \cdots + \frac{(10 - 7.659)^2}{7.659}$$
$$= 10.84$$

The number of degrees of freedom has been reduced to 6, so that from the tables giving the critical values of chi-square (Table C) we find that:

$$\chi_{0.10}^2 (\text{df} = 6) = 10.64$$
$$\chi_{0.05}^2 (\text{df} = 6) = 12.59$$

i.e. the observed value falls between these two so that:

$$0.05 < P < 0.10$$

Thus the null hypothesis would be accepted and it would be concluded that smoking habits are independent of age.

If chi-square is calculated for the original data in this example, where 42% of the expected values were below 5, a value of 18.90 at 9 degrees of freedom is obtained. Reference to the table shows that *P* is less than 0.05 and very close to 0.025 and thus, at the 5% level of significance, the null hypothesis would have been rejected in favour of the alternative, and it would have been concluded that the proportions were not all equal, or that smoking habits *are* dependent on age. This is, of course, not a valid test.

In general, the way in which data are to be analysed should be decided before the data are collected. If insufficient data is gathered, it may well transpire that a satisfactory chi-square test cannot be performed.

Remember that if you decide to work at the 5% level of significance, this means that you are prepared to accept a 5% chance of wrongly rejecting the null hypothesis in favour of the experimental hypothesis.

A 2 × 2 contingency table

If a contingency table only contains two rows and two columns (a 2 × 2 table), and thus only 1 degree of freedom, chi-square is usually calculated in a slightly different way, although, once again, opinions are divided regarding the necessity of such a variation. In this case chi-square is calculated as follows:

$$\chi_0^2 = \sum \frac{(|O - E| - 0.5)^2}{E} \tag{7.2}$$

where $|O - E|$ is the 'modulus' of the difference between the observed and expected values, i.e. the magnitude of the difference, irrespective of the sign. This is known as the 'Yates continuity correction' and is applied because the chi-square statistic, as defined, only approximates to the continuous chi-square distribution since we are concerned with discrete cell frequencies. If the expected cell frequencies are large, however, the difference between the corrected and uncorrected value of chi-square is small and the correction becomes less important.

In the case of a 2 × 2 table, it is possible to conduct either a directional or non-directional test. To avoid confusion it is better not to refer to these as two-tailed or one-tailed tests because only one tail of the distribution curve is considered. For a directional test, the P value obtained from the table of critical values of χ^2 (Table C) is halved.

The following example illustrates this point.

Example 7.4

An experiment was conducted to determine whether the response to a simple question requiring a yes/no answer was independent of the sex of the respondent. The following data were collected:

	Female	Male
Yes	20	13
No	6	13

The equal numbers in the second column have been included deliberately to illustrate the nature of a directional chi-square test.

Consider the possible experimental hypotheses:

—the proportion of females who answered 'yes' was *different* from the males; or

—the proportion of females who answered 'yes' was *greater* than the males.

In the first case above the experimental hypothesis is:

$$H_1: \ p_F \neq p_M$$

and in the second:

$$H_1: \ p_F > p_M$$

where p represents the proportion who answer 'yes'.

Note that it is only possible to perform a directional test in the case of a 2×2 table and not with larger tables because, in general, proportions with more than two components cannot be quantified relative to each other in the same way. The expected values can now be calculated in the usual way:

	Female	Male	Total
Yes	20 (16.50)	13 (16.50)	33
No	6 (9.50)	13 (9.50)	19
Total	26	26	52

and hence chi-square, including the Yates correction, may be calculated:

$$\chi_0^2 = \frac{(|20 - 16.50| - 0.5)^2}{16.50} + \cdots + \frac{(|13 - 9.50| - 0.5)^2}{9.50}$$

$$= 2.99$$

If the proportions in the female group had been 6:20 rather than 20:6, the calculated value of chi-square would have been exactly the same. This is only the case, of course, because the male group is equally divided 13:13. These numbers have been chosen to illustrate the general point showing the two possible 'directions'. The same principle applies if the proportions in the second column are not equal, but, in that case, the chi-square value would not be exactly the same if the ratio in the second column is inverted.

Reference to the tables at 1 degree of freedom shows:

$$\chi_{0.05}^2 = 3.84$$
$$\chi_{0.10}^2 = 2.71$$

which refers to a normal non-directional alternative hypothesis which asserts that the proportion saying 'yes' is different for male and female respondents. Equally, it could be put the other way round asserting that the proportion of males (or females) is different in the group saying 'yes' and the group saying 'no'. Thus for a non-directional test:

$$0.05 < P < 0.10$$

This range includes both the situation where the proportion in the female group who answer 'yes' compared with those who answer 'no' is 20:6 and also where it is 6:20. So, if we wish to demonstrate that the proportion of females who answer 'yes' is greater than for males, we would use a directional test and postulate the second of the two possible experimental hypotheses, whereupon the P value is halved, i.e. we are ignoring the possibility that the proportion could be 6 : 20 because it is not thought to be feasible. We would therefore conclude that:

$$0.025 < P < 0.05$$

The null hypothesis is, of course, the same in either case, i.e.

$$H_0: p_F = p_M$$

Note that in the above example, the expected frequencies in each column are the same because each contains the same total.

Summary

THE CHI-SQUARE TEST involves entering all actual observed frequencies into the table. They must not be converted to percentages because the value of chi-square is very much dependent on the sample size. In the case of the above example when $\chi^2 = 2.99$, if the observed frequencies are all multiplied by 10 then $\chi^2 = 39.5$, and the probability that this latter value will occur by chance is virtually zero.

LOW EXPECTED FREQUENCIES. No more than 20% of cells should have expected frequencies less than 5, which in the case of a 2×2 table means that there should be none less than 5. If expected frequencies are below 5, the Fisher–Irwin exact test may be applied. A discussion of this test is beyond the scope of this text, but an example of its application may be found, if required, in *Statistical Methods in Laboratory Medicine* by Paul Strike (Butterworth–Heinemann 1991). No cells should have an expected frequency less than unity.

Exercises for Chapter 7

Exercise 7.1

A group, selected at random, comprising several categories of therapists, was asked a particular question to which the answers 'yes', 'no' or 'don't know' were recorded with the following frequencies:

	Therapist		
	Occupational	Physio-	Speech
Yes	9	4	4
No	7	9	5
Don't know	6	6	14

Is the response independent of the category of the respondent?

Exercise 7.2

The frequency of visits by patients to a physiotherapist were categorized according to age as follows:

		Age group			
		20–29	30–39	40–49	50–59
Number of visits	<3	5	14	12	9
	3–5	2	6	7	2
	>5	3	5	11	8

Can it be concluded that the frequency is independent of age?

Exercise 7.3

An investigation was carried out to compare two treatments for a particular problem, with and without traction. The following data were collected:

	Traction	No traction
No improvement	8	3
Improvement	14	23

Is the difference between the two treatments significant at the 5% level?

Exercise 7.4

A group of 400 patients were categorized according to their physical build and mental state with the following results:

	Fat	Normal	Thin
Normal	82	140	78
Neurotic	7	34	16
Psychotic	8	28	7

Are we able to conclude that the mental state is independent of physical stature?

Exercise 7.5

In a survey of eight-year-old children, it was found that nine out of 174 who were born prematurely and five out of 295 who had a normal birth, suffered with myopia.

(a) Calculate the percentage of myopic children in each category.
(b) Can it be concluded that the incidence of myopia is independent of the nature of the birth?
(c) Can it be concluded that a greater percentage of prematurely born children suffer with myopia?

8

A Comparison of More than Two Means

Contents
—Analysis of variance (ANOVA): why is this necessary?
—The principles behind ANOVA.
—The comparison of variances using the F-test and the one-way ANOVA.
—ANOVA with repeated measures.

Introduction

In this chapter, we shall consider the basic principles behind 'analysis of variance', generally referred to as ANOVA, and the reasons why such a procedure is necessary.

In order to compare the means of two samples, a t-test is employed. However, if there are more than two samples, several t-tests comparing them in pairs is not a satisfactory solution to the problem for two reasons. Firstly, in order to compare four sample means in pairs, six t-tests would need to be performed, because there are six different ways of selecting two samples from four. For six samples, 15 tests would be required.

It can be shown that the number of different ways of selecting x objects from a total of n, which is known as a 'combination' and is represented by ^nC_x, may be calculated as follows:

$$^nC_x = \frac{n!}{n!\,(n-x)!}$$

where $n! = $ 'factorial n', i.e. $n(n-1)(n-2)\ldots 1$. For example, if there are four samples $(n=4)$ and we wish to select them in pairs $(x=2)$, then:

$$n! = 4! = 4 \times 3 \times 2 \times 1$$

and

$$x! = 2! = 2 \times 1$$

$$^nC_x = \frac{4!}{2!\,(4-2)!} = 6$$

Secondly, the probability of committing what is known as a Type I error, that is, rejecting the null hypothesis when it is true, becomes unacceptably higher. This can be seen by the following argument.

If working at the 5% level of significance, i.e. $\alpha = 0.05$, in a single t-test, this represents the probability of rejecting the null hypothesis when it is actually true, because, of course, this is the probability that the observed value of t will exceed the critical value, with the appropriate number of degrees of freedom by chance.

If the probability of wrongly rejecting the hypothesis is 0.05, then the probability of correctly rejecting it is 0.95, for a single test. Thus, for six tests, the probability of correctly rejecting the hypothesis in all six tests is $(0.95)^6$, i.e. 0.74, which is unacceptably low.

It is important to understand the principles behind the way in which the ANOVA works, which, in fact, are quite simple.

It is also important to remember that certain assumptions are made when performing an ANOVA, namely, (i) that the data follow, at least approximately, a normal distribution, and (ii) that the variances of the different samples are not significantly different from each other.

Analysis of variance—principles

In Chapter 5 we saw that the standard error of the mean $(s_{\bar{x}})$, that is, the standard deviation of the means of a number of samples taken from the same population, is given by $s/\sqrt{n}$, where n is the size of the sample, and s is the standard deviation determined from the sample, which is, of course, an estimate of the population value, i.e.

$$s_{\bar{x}} = \frac{s}{\sqrt{n}}$$

$$\text{or} \quad s_{\bar{x}}^2 = \frac{s^2}{n}$$

(8.1)

The basic principle behind the ANOVA technique is that the variance of the data within the groups (samples) is estimated by two different methods, the first, the 'between-group variance' is calculated from the variability of the sample means, and is thus dependent on any differences between them, and the 'within-group variance' which is a 'pooled estimate of the variance' similar to that employed in the two sample t-test, which, you will remember, is simply an average variance 'weighted' according to the number of degrees of freedom of each sample.

The two values of the variance are compared using the F-test (see later in this chapter) and if the between-group variance is significantly larger than the within-group variance, this can only be because the means of the various samples are significantly different from each other. If the two variance estimates are shown to be not significantly different, we conclude that the effect of the variability of the means is not significant, that is, the means are not significantly different from each other. If, however, the within-group variance is the larger, this can only be the result of chance, so we need proceed no further and accept the null hypothesis that the means are not significantly different from each other.

These two methods of estimating the variance are now considered in a little more detail.

The between-group variance

The value of the standard error of the mean may be obtained by simply determining the mean of each sample and calculating the standard deviation of these means. The standard deviation of the data within the groups may be estimated from this by rearranging the equation. In the context of the ANOVA, this is referred to as the between-group variance estimate, s_b^2

$$s^2 = s_b^2 = ns_{\bar{x}}^2 \tag{8.2}$$

This method of calculating the between-group variance may only be used if all the samples are the same size (n). A more general approach is considered later in this chapter.

The within-group variance

The alternative estimate of the variance of the data may be obtained as a 'pooled estimate' which, as was indicated above, is calculated in exactly the same way as in the case of the two sample t-test, i.e. it is an average variance, 'weighted' according to the size, or, more strictly, number of degrees of freedom in each sample, and is referred to as the within-group variance estimate, s_w^2, i.e.

$$s^2 = s_w^2 = \frac{(n_A - 1)s_A^2 + (n_B - 1)s_B^2 + \cdots + (n_n - 1)s_n^2}{(n_A - 1) + (n_B - 1) + \cdots + (n_n - 1)} \tag{8.3}$$

Thus, the between-group variance estimate *is* dependent on variability between the means, and the within-group variance estimate *is not* dependent on any variability between the means. So that if no significant difference exists between the two variance estimates, then it can be concluded that no significant difference exists between the sample means. This can be tested with an F-test, which is now described.

This method of calculating the within-group variance is included to illustrate the principle of the calculation. However, it is not necessary for the samples to be all the same size and a more general method, which is usually used is described later in this chapter.

The F-test

The F-test is a general test used to compare variances, or standard deviations, and is not specific to the ANOVA, but is incidental to it, so the ANOVA should not be referred to as an F-test. The F-test will first be considered simply as a test to compare variances, and not as part of the ANOVA procedure.

The statistic, F, is defined:

$$F(df_A, df_B) = \left(\frac{s_A/\sigma_A}{s_B/\sigma_B} \right)^2 = \left(\frac{s_A^2/\sigma_A^2}{s_B^2/\sigma_B^2} \right) \qquad (8.4)$$

where:

s_A and $s_B =$ the standard deviations of samples A and B,
σ_A and $\sigma_B =$ the standard deviations of the populations from which they were taken.

Note that the number of degrees of freedom of each sample must be quoted.

Since the null hypothesis is that there is no difference between the population values of the two variances, i.e.

$$H_0: \quad \sigma_A^2 = \sigma_B^2$$

the definition of the statistic F, for the purposes of the test becomes:

$$F(df_A, df_B) = \frac{s_A^2}{s_B^2} \qquad (8.5)$$

The F- and chi-square distributions are both asymmetric and similar in shape. The F-distribution, however, is dependent on the number of degrees of freedom of both samples, and therefore a separate table is necessary for each significance level. Table D in Appendix VI gives the values of F which are significant at 5%, 2.5% and 1%, respectively. For convenience, the tables normally only give probabilities for values of F greater than unity, and since the samples are designated A and B arbitrarily, F is calculated by dividing the larger variance estimate by the smaller. The following example illustrates the use of the F-test to compare variances. In this case, therefore, it is a comparison of precision.

Example 8.1

It is required to compare the precision of two observers in measuring heart rate. For this purpose six measurements (beats/min) were taken on a resting subject by each of two observers, A and B. One measurement by observer B was discarded because it was obviously in error.

The unequal sample sizes have been chosen deliberately to illustrate the nature of the non-directional test, but, of course, they may equally well both be the same size.

Observer A	77	77	79	79	78	79
Observer B	74	76	78	76	79	

Note that these data represent two statistical samples. The population in each case would be an infinite number of observations.

The relevant hypotheses are:

$$H_0: \ \sigma_A = \sigma_B \quad \text{or} \quad \sigma_A^2 = \sigma_B^2$$
$$H_1: \ \sigma_A \neq \sigma_B \quad \quad \ \ \sigma_A^2 \neq \sigma_B^2$$

Using a hand calculator, the standard deviations of the two samples, and hence F, may be determined. As before, F_0 represents the observed value of F and remember that it is calculated, for convenience, so that F is greater than unity.

$$s_A = 0.983 \quad s_B = 1.949$$

$$F_0(5, 4) = \left(\frac{s_B^2}{s_A^2} \right) = \frac{1.949^2}{0.983^2} = 3.93$$

Working at a 5% level of significance for a non-directional or two-way test, the critical value of F at the 2.5% level is required. This is obtained from Table D, where the number of degrees of freedom for the larger variance estimate, in this case 5, for sample A is represented across the top of the table, and for the smaller, 4, down the left-hand side. From the table:

$$F_{0.025}(5, 4) = 9.36$$

We see also that:

$$F_{0.025}(4, 5) = 7.39$$

Thus if $s_B > s_A$ the difference is said to be significant if $F_0(5, 4)$, that is the observed value of F, exceeds 9.36. If $s_A > s_B$ the difference is significant if $F_0(4, 5)$ exceeds 7.39.

In this case the former critical value of F is appropriate because $s_B > s_A$ and since the observed value, 3.93, is less than the critical value, 9.36, the null hypothesis is accepted and it is concluded that there is no significant difference between the variances, i.e. the precision of the measurements taken by the two observers at the 5% level. In other words there is insufficient evidence at this level to reject the null hypothesis, it is therefore accepted.

The fact that the critical values at the 5% level for $F(5, 4)$ and $F(4, 5)$ are not the same is, of course, a result of the difference in the sample sizes.

Since the tables only quote values of F greater than unity, it is not possible to consider both tails of the $F_{0.025}(5, 4)$ distribution. The above procedure shows the approach to the non-directional or two-way test.

Analysis of variance

The discussion at the beginning of this chapter was intended to give an insight into the nature of the principles behind the ANOVA. Although it is perfectly possible to determine the 'between-group variance' by determining the variance of the sample means, which is then multiplied by the number of observations in each sample (provided they are all the same size), and similarly, the 'within-group variance' may be calculated as a 'pooled average', this is, as was mentioned above, not the usual approach. The reason for this is that a standard approach which is applicable to the various forms of ANOVA is used, and the above procedure is only appropriate for the simplest one-way ANOVA, that is, where only a single independent variable is involved and all the samples are the same size.

Assumptions

We should remember that a number of assumptions are made when conducting an analysis of variance.

—The data should, in principle, follow, at least approximately, a normal distribution. The procedure is, however, quite 'robust', i.e. it is not influenced a great deal by departures from normality.
—The variances of the samples should not be significantly different from each other.

The general procedures for the ANOVA are now described in some detail.

Care must be taken to avoid confusion because the term 'sum of the squares' is used to refer to the sum of the squares of various differences between variables and means, e.g. the 'total sum of the squares' (SST) and the 'sum of the squares of the columns' (SSC) are given, together with rearranged forms to make the calculation a little more simple:

$$SST = \sum (x - \bar{G})^2$$
$$= \sum x^2 - \frac{G^2}{N} \qquad (8.6)$$

and

$$SSC = \sum n(\bar{x} - \bar{G})^2$$
$$= \sum \frac{T^2}{n} - \frac{G^2}{N} \qquad (8.7)$$

where:

$\sum x^2 = x_1^2 + x_2^2 + x_3^2 + \cdots + x_N^2,$
$\bar{G}$ = the 'grand mean', i.e. the mean of all the data,
G = the 'grand sum', i.e. the sum of all the data,
T = the sum of each column,
n = the number of observations in each column,
N = the total number of observations.

We can see that the 'total sum of the squares' is a measure of the variability of the observations about the 'grand mean', and the 'sum of the squares of the columns' is a measure of the variability within the columns estimated from the variability of the column means (i.e. the sample means) about the 'grand mean'. In the case of the latter, n appears in the equation because of the relationship between the variance of the data, which is being estimated, and the variance of the column means (see Equation 8.2).

The advantage of using the sums of the squares as a measure of variability is that they can be added and subtracted from each other, thus indicating the various contributions to the total variability. On the other hand, in the case of the 'mean sums of the squares', or the variances, this, in general, cannot be done.

For the purposes of the ANOVA we also require the 'sum of the squares of the error' (SSE). The SST is a measure of the total variability, and the SSC is a measure of the variability of the data estimated from the variability of the means of the columns, i.e. the samples. The SSE, which is sometimes referred to as the 'residual sum of the squares', is a measure of the variability within the samples which is *independent* of any variability in the sample means and is obtained by subtracting SSC from SST, i.e.

$$\text{SSE} = \text{SST} - \text{SSC} \tag{8.8}$$

Each is then divided by the number of degrees of freedom associated with the particular variability to obtain the 'mean sum of the squares' (MS) from which F is calculated.

Variance or the mean sum of the squares

Note that in the context of the ANOVA, the sum of the squares divided by the number of degrees of freedom, which is actually a variance, is normally referred to as 'the mean sum of the squares', or MS. This is because the variability does not refer to the data as a whole, but to particular aspects of the data, e.g. the column means.

The calculations are usually set out as follows ($k =$ the number of columns):

Source of variation	SS	DF	MS	$F(k-1, N-k)$
Columns	SSC	$k-1$	$\text{SSC}/(k-1)$ $= \text{MSC}$	MSC/MSE
Error	SSE	$N-k$	$\text{SSE}/(N-k)$ $= \text{MSE}$	
Total	SST	$N-1$		

If the SST is divided by the total number of degrees of freedom $(N - 1)$, we have the variance of the data as a whole. However, in the ANOVA the SST is calculated simply as a step towards obtaining SSE.

The number of degrees of freedom associated with SSC is $(k - 1)$ because it is estimated from the means of k columns, and for the SSE, it is simply the difference $[(N - 1) - (k - 1)]$, i.e. $(N - k)$, or $(n - 1)$ for each column exactly as in the case of the 'pooled' estimate of the variance.

We can see that MSC and MSE are simply the between-group and within-group variance considered earlier in this chapter (s_b^2 and s_w^2 respectively).

The following example illustrates a simple one-way ANOVA, that is, there is a single independent variable only. In other words, there is only a single factor that is changed under the control of the experimenter, in this case, it is the use of a different method of measuring the heart rate. The 'response variable' is the measured heart rate by each method.

Example 8.2

Consider again the data in Example 8.1. They are required to compare, this time for reliability, the two methods of measuring heart rate, together with two additional methods. The data already collected are to be used together with data from the the additional measurements, taken, of course, at the same time and on the same resting subject. The following results were obtained:

Method			
A	B	C	D
77	74	76	75
77	76	80	73
79	78	77	71
79	76	76	74
78	79	78	74
79		78	76

Column sum $(T) = 469$ 383   465   443
Grand sum $(G) = 469\ +\ 383\ +\ 465\ +\ 449 = 1,760$
Sample size $(n) =\quad 6\qquad 5\qquad 6\qquad 6$

The appropriate hypotheses, which, it should be stressed, are in terms of the means and not the variances, are:

$$H_0: \mu_1 = \mu_2 = \mu_3 = \mu_4$$

$$H_1: \text{not all means are equal}$$

Note that the alternative hypothesis should *not* be written:

$$H_1: \mu_1 \neq \mu_2 \neq \mu_3 \neq \mu_4$$

The various 'sums of the squares' may now be calculated using Equations 8.6, 8.7 and 8.8:

$$SST = \sum X^2 - \frac{G^2}{N}$$

$$= (77^2 + 77^2 + 79^2 + \cdots + 74^2 + 76^2) - \frac{1,760^2}{23}$$

$$= 134,790 - 134,678.26$$

$$= 111.74$$

Note that this calculation involves subtracting one large number from another and the difference between the two is small, therefore it is advisable to maintain a large number of significant figures until the final result is obtained.

$$SSC = \sum \frac{T^2}{n} - \frac{G^2}{N}$$

$$= \left(\frac{469^2}{6} + \frac{383^2}{5} + \frac{465^2}{6} + \frac{443^2}{6} \right) - \frac{1,760^2}{23}$$

$$= 134,743.63 - 134,678.26$$

$$= 65.37$$

$$SSC = SST - SSC = 111.74 - 65.37 = 46.37$$

The ANOVA table can now be constructed:

Source of variation	SS	df	MS	F
Column means	65.37	3	12.79	8.93
Error	46.37	19	2.44	
Total	111.74	22		

Remember that there are 3 degrees of freedom associated with the variability of the column means, because there are four columns, and there are 22 degrees of freedom associated with the total sum of the squares because there are 23 observations altogether. The number of degrees of freedom associated with the 'error' or 'residual' is the difference between the two, or, recalling that this represents a 'pooled' estimate of the variance, there are $(n - 1)$ degrees of freedom for each column (sample), i.e. $(5 + 4 + 5 + 5) = 19$.

The number of degrees of freedom (df) for each source of variation is shown in the ANOVA table. Consulting the tables for the F distribution for the critical value of F at 1% (Table D) at 3 and 19 degrees of freedom we find:

$$F_{0.01}(3, 19) = 5.01$$

The ANOVA always requires a one-way test because, if there is a significant difference between the variance estimates, we expect the between-group variance, that is the variance estimated from the column means, to be larger than the within-group variance, i.e. the 'error variance', above. The reason for this is that the former is dependent on variability between the sample means and the latter is not. As a consequence, in the case of an ANOVA, if a value for F, which is always calculated as MSC/MSE, is obtained which is less than unity, we would immediately accept the null hypothesis because the difference between the variance estimates can only be by random chance.

Referring again to the tabulated values for F, remember that this means that there is only a 1% probability that F will take a value of 5.01, or larger, by chance alone. Thus, since the observed value is 8.93, which is considerably greater than this, the probability that it has occurred by chance is a good deal less than 1%, so the null hypothesis may be rejected with much less than a 1% chance that we are wrong, i.e.

$$P < 0.01$$

Thus, we would conclude that the various methods do *not* all yield the same results, or, at least one mean is significantly different from the others at the 1% level.

It is worth noting that, if there are only two samples, exactly the same conclusion will be reached if either an independent sample *t*-test with a pooled estimate of the standard deviation or an ANOVA is performed.

Further investigation of the column means

The conclusion reached in the above example of an ANOVA is that at least one of the sets of measurements has a significantly different mean from the rest, but it tells us no more than that. More information may be obtained by calculating the 'least significant difference' between the means using what is often referred to as a 'protected *t*-test'. The sample statistic in this case is the difference between two means, the variance of which, it can be shown, is given by:

$$\text{var}(\bar{x} - \bar{x}') = s_w^2\left(\frac{1}{n} + \frac{1}{n'}\right) \qquad (8.9)$$

where s_w^2 is the estimate of the within-group variance, or MS(Error), i.e. the mean sum of the squares and is based on $(N - k)$ degrees of freedom. Thus the standard error of this difference:

$$\text{SE}(\bar{x} - \bar{x}') = s_w\sqrt{\frac{1}{n} + \frac{1}{n'}} \qquad (8.10)$$

By rearranging Equation 6.1, the least difference between two means which is significant at the 5% level may be calculated:

$$(\bar{x} - \bar{x}') = t_{0.025}s_w\sqrt{\frac{1}{n} + \frac{1}{n'}} \qquad (8.11)$$

where $t_{0.025}$ is the value of t with the number of degrees of freedom associated with the error term, i.e. $(N - k)$, or 19. Reference to Table B shows, for one tail, this to be 2.093. The sizes of the two samples with which we are concerned in considering the significance of the difference between the means are represented by n and n'.

Thus, in the above example, for two samples of dissimilar sizes, the least significant difference is given by:

$$(\bar{x} - \bar{x}') = 2.093\sqrt{2.44}\sqrt{\frac{1}{5} + \frac{1}{6}}$$

$$= 2.0 \tag{8.12}$$

and between two of the same size:

$$(\bar{x} - \bar{x}') = 2.093\sqrt{2.44}\sqrt{\frac{1}{6} + \frac{1}{6}}$$

$$= 1.9 \tag{8.13}$$

For the next step, the means are arranged in order of magnitude and the differences between them noted:

$\bar{x}_D$	$<$	$\bar{x}_B$	$<$	$\bar{x}_C$	$<$	$\bar{x}_A$
$(n = 6)$		$(n = 5)$		$(n = 6)$		$(n = 6)$
73.8		76.6		77.5		78.2

| 2.8 | 0.9 | 0.7 |

We can see from Equation 12 that for the means of samples D and B, being of size 6 and 5 respectively, the least significant difference is 2.0. Similarly for samples B and C. For samples C and A, however, both being of size 6 we can see, referring to Equation 8.13, that the least significant difference is 1.9. Looking at the differences we see that:

$$(\bar{x}_B - \bar{x}_D) > 2.0$$

but

$$(\bar{x}_C - \bar{x}_B) < 2.0$$
$$(\bar{x}_A - \bar{x}_C) < 1.9$$

i.e. samples B, C and A are not significantly different from each other, but sample D is significantly different from the other three. This result may be represented:

$$\underline{\mu_D} \quad \underline{\mu_B \quad \mu_C \quad \mu_A}$$

We would therefore conclude that method D yields a result which is significantly different from the other three, which are not significantly different from each other.

You will no doubt realize that the above treatment really amounts to a multiple t-test, which, as was stated at the beginning of this chapter, is not an appropriate approach to the problem of comparing more than two sample means. However, in this case the null hypothesis has already been rejected, and the least significant difference is calculated using the 'error (within-group) variance' which compensates to some extent, and the value of t that is used is based on $(N - k)$ degrees of freedom. This method does tend to slightly overestimate the number of significant differences, but it has the advantage of being simple and, for this reason, is often used rather than some of the more complex methods that are available.

Analysis of variance with repeated measures

This is the ANOVA equivalent of a related, or paired sample t-test. In the case of the t-test we have, for each subject, only two conditions under which measurements are taken, i.e. repeated, whereas in the case of the ANOVA, we have repeated measures, or observations, on each subject under more than two conditions.

Let us refer back to Example 8.2 but consider a rather changed situation where the heart rate was measured using the four distinct methods but on several *different* subjects. In this case, if we wish to compare the methods of measurement, it is necessary to eliminate any variability resulting from the difference in the actual heart rate of each subject.

Basically this is a two-way ANOVA because there are two independent variables, namely (i) the change in the measuring devices, and (ii) the different subjects.

The sums of the squares are calculated in exactly the same way as in the case of the one-way ANOVA except in this case the sum of the squares of the columns (SSC) is a measure of the variability between the methods, and the sum of the squares of the rows (SSR) is a measure of the variability of the heart rate between subjects.

Consider the following example.

Example 8.3

Five different subjects were asked to relax for 15 minutes and then the heart rate of each was measured by the four different methods. The following data were collected:

| Subject | Method | | | | T_r |
	I	II	III	IV	
A	71	68	65	70	274
B	74	68	70	71	283
C	78	79	78	73	308
D	76	75	74	72	297
E	74	74	73	72	293
T_k	373	364	360	358	1,455

where:
T_k = the column total
T_r = the row total
G = the grand total
    = 1,455
N = the total number of observations
    = 20

The null and alternative hypotheses are, as previously:

$$H_0: \mu_1 = \mu_2 = \mu_3 = \mu_4$$

$$H_1: \text{not all means are equal}$$

where μ_1 to μ_4 are the means of columns 1 to 4 respectively.

The various sums of the squares may now be calculated. Firstly the total sum of the squares (Equation 8.6):

$$SST = \sum x^2 - \frac{G^2}{N}$$
$$= (71^2 + 74^2 + 78^2 + \cdots + 72^2 + 72^2) - \frac{1,455^2}{20}$$
$$= 106,095 - 105,851.25$$
$$= 243.75$$

The sum of the squares for the variation between the methods of measurement, that is the variability of the column means, is calculated exactly as in the case of the one way ANOVA (Equation 8.7):

$$SSC = \sum \frac{T_k^2}{n_r} - \frac{G^2}{N}$$
$$= \left(\frac{343^2}{5} + \frac{364^2}{5} + \frac{360^2}{5} + \frac{358^2}{5}\right) - \frac{1,455^2}{20}$$
$$= 105,877.80 - 105,851.25$$
$$= 26.55$$

where n_r is the number of rows, or the number of observations in each column.

The variability resulting from the fact that measurements have been taken on different subjects who, of course, would not be expected to have the same heart rate, is evaluated in terms of the sum of the squares of the rows, i.e. the variability of the row means:

$$SSR = \sum \frac{T_r^2}{n_k} - \frac{G^2}{N} \tag{8.14}$$

where n_k is the number of columns, or the number of observations in each row.

$$SSR = \left(\frac{274^2}{4} + \frac{283^2}{4} + \cdots + \frac{308^2}{4} + \frac{297^2}{4} + \frac{293^2}{4}\right) - \frac{1,455^2}{20}$$
$$= 106,021.75 - 105,851.25$$
$$= 170.50$$

Note that in both of the above, that is SSC and SSR, the first term is the summation of the square of the column or row totals, respectively, divided by the number of observations making that total, i.e. the number of rows (n_r) in the case of SSC and the number of columns (n_k) in the case of SSR.

As before, in the case of the simple one-way ANOVA, the variation resulting from random error is obtained by subtraction.

$$SSE = SST - SSC - SSR$$
$$= 243.75 - 26.55 - 170.50$$
$$= 46.70$$

The ANOVA table may now be constructed:

Source of variation	SS	df	MS	F
Methods (columns)	26.55	3	8.85	$8.85/3.89 = 2.28$
Subjects (rows)	170.50	4	(42.63)	$(42.63/3.89 = 10.96)$
Error	46.70	12	3.89	
Total	243.75	19		

The mean sum of the squares of the rows and the associated F value are included in brackets because these are not required in the case of a one-way ANOVA with repeated measures, but are included for completeness. If we wished also to compare the pulse rates of the different subjects, this value of F would enable us to do so.

The sum of the squares associated with the column means is, of course, a measure of the variability in methods of measurement and the sum of the squares associated with the row means is a measure of variability in the heart rates of the different subjects. The latter is calculated simply so that it may be eliminated, but needs to be determined in order to obtain a value for the random error effect.

The value of F above is calculated as MS(Column means)/MS(Error), i.e. 8.85/3.89 $=$ 2.28 with 3 and 12 degrees of freedom. Reference to Table D shows that at the 5% level:

$$F_{0.05}(3, \ 12) = 3.49$$

The observed value, 2.28, is less than the critical value, 3.49. Remember that the larger the observed value of F, the less likely it is that it has occurred by chance and the more likely that there is a real difference between the variances. Conversely, of course, this means that if the value of F is small, it is unlikely that a real difference exists. In this case F is smaller than the critical value, that is the value that we would expect to be exceeded by random chance if the null hypothesis is true. Therefore the conclusion is that the null hypothesis is accepted, i.e. the differences in the results obtained by the various heart rate measuring methods are not significant at the 5% level.

Although not of importance here, we can see that the value of F relating to the variability between subjects, i.e. of the row means, MS(Row means)/MS(Error) is 10.96. This value, at 4 and 12 degrees of freedom, is well above the value at the 5% level of significance, and, we can see from Table D, it is above 5.41, the critical value at 1%, i.e. $P < 0.01$. This is not really surprising, because we would not expect different subjects to have the same resting heart rate.

Summary

ANALYSIS OF VARIANCE is employed if it is necessary to compare the means of more than two samples, in which case the use of multiple t-tests is not a satisfactory approach. In such a procedure, the variance of the data is estimated in two ways, one that is dependent on the variability of the sample means (between-group variance) and one that is not (the within-group, error or residual variance). If the former is found to be significantly larger than the latter, using the F-test, then the cause of this must be variability of the sample means, which, it is then concluded, must be significantly different from each other.

If the error variance is larger than the between-group variance, i.e. F is less than unity, this can only result from random effects and the null hypothesis must be accepted. Remember that if the null hypothesis is true ($H_0: \sigma_w^2 = \sigma_b^2$) the 'expected' value of F will be unity, although it will, of course, vary from this by random chance. There is thus a 50% probability that $F > 1.0$ and a 50% probability that $F < 1.0$.

TWO-WAY ANOVA is used if two independent variables are involved or repeated observations, or measures as they are often called, are taken. In the latter case, the variability between subjects may thus be eliminated.

Exercises for Chapter 8

Exercise 8.1

The following data were collected from four samples:

A	B	C	D
18	28	23	21
21	30	29	23
24	26	28	27
18	32	30	21
28	31	25	20

(a) Perform an analysis of variance (ANOVA) to determine whether there is a significant difference between the means of the populations from which the above samples have been taken.

(b) Why would a series of t-tests between pairs of samples be an unsatisfactory way of approaching the problem? *If* this were done, how many t-tests would be required?

(c) Calculate the least significant difference between the means and hence consider whether any further information about the relationships may be obtained.

Exercise 8.2

Eight patients suffering from migraine were treated by an osteopath and asked to record the number of hours per week that they suffered headaches. The first two weeks were without treatment and the subsequent three weeks were recorded each after one treatment session. The following data were collected:

	Week				
	1	2	3	4	5
Mr A	25	21	20	18	20
Mr B	23	17	25	15	16
Mrs C	18	19	22	17	11
Miss D	27	20	23	24	19
Mr E	24	26	18	25	18
Mr F	25	27	17	17	16
Mrs G	26	20	20	19	19
Mrs H	20	26	20	17	18

Can it be concluded that the duration of headaches per week had altered as a result of the treatment?

Exercise 8.3

A physiotherapist in a city gymnasium performed an experiment to compare the systolic blood pressure of members from different professions. The following data were collected:

Profession			
A	B	C	D
118	120	124	138
119	115	122	142
103	141	152	122
137	134	137	155
142	110	113	145
112	127	136	149
144	128	–	123
–	115	–	152

Is there a significant difference between the means of the four samples at the 5% level?

Exercise 8.4

A group of 32 therapists, matched for qualifications and experience, attended a short course and, for the purpose of assessing different teaching methods, were assigned, quite randomly, to four groups of eight individuals. Each group was taught by a different method (A, B, C and D) and assessed at the end of the course. The following marks were recorded:

Group			
A	B	C	D
73	58	77	53
59	69	78	55
73	52	58	53
71	65	75	49
68	62	68	69
65	57	64	69
76	54	58	53
58	61	75	51

Test the hypothesis that the teaching methods are equally effective. What further information may be obtained by employing a protected t-test?

Exercise 8.5

An experiment was conducted to compare the power grip strength (kg) of male subjects in four different age groups with the following results:

Age range			
A 20–29	B 30–39	C 40–49	D 50–59
66	68	55	55
51	62	60	35
47	57	58	49
55	60	52	45
50	49	49	57
54	59	49	43
47	55	54	44
68	53	58	46

(a) Test the hypothesis that at least one of the means is significantly different from the others at the 5% level.
(b) Use the protected t-test to determine whether one particular mean is significantly smaller or larger than the rest.

Exercise 8.6

An experiment was conducted to determine whether a significant difference existed in the strength of the quadriceps measured at hip flex 90°, 45° and 0° for both the dominant and the non-dominant leg. The following data were collected from 11 subjects:

Dominant leg			Non-dominant leg		
90°	45°	0°	90°	45°	0°
13	13	14	14	15	16
22	21	25	20	19	20
14	14	13	12	13	11
15	17	15	15	14	14
15	17	19	16	16	16
18	17	15	16	15	13
17	15	16	12	11	14
16	13	14	16	12	13
14	13	12	14	14	13
14	13	13	17	16	13
24	18	20	22	20	18

Perform two analyses of variance to test the hypothesis that, at the 5% level, there is not a significant difference between the strength of the quadriceps at different angles (i) in the dominant, and (ii) in the non-dominant leg.

Exercise 8.7

Use the data given in Exercise 8.6 above and compare the average strength of the quadriceps at the three angles for the dominant leg with the average for the non-dominant leg.

Note: this may be tested using either a paired sample t-test or analysis of variance. Although there are only two samples, the latter will yield exactly the same result. It is a useful exercise to carry out both procedures to confirm this.

9

Non-parametric Tests

Contents
—The Mann–Whitney or Wilcoxon rank-sum test.
—The Wilcoxon matched-pair signed-ranks test.
—The Kruskal–Wallis non-parametric ANOVA.
—The Friedman non-parametric one-way ANOVA with repeated measures.

Introduction

In general, the statistical tests which have been considered in previous chapters have involved the estimation of parameters associated with the frequency distributions of the populations from which the samples were taken. For example, the t-test is concerned with the standard deviations and the means of samples, which are statistics, and are estimates of the corresponding population values, which are parameters. In addition, the assumption is made that the distribution is, at least approximately, normal. Thus, such procedures are known as 'parametric tests' and, in general, are used in the case of interval, or ratio data (see Chapter 1).

Parametric and non-parametric tests

In this chapter some tests which require no such assumption are described. They may be used in the case of nominal or ordinal data, or in the case of interval or ratio data when no assumption can be made about the population probability distribution. The tests are therefore valid no matter what form the distribution may take and for this reason are often referred to as 'distribution-free' or 'non-parametric' tests.

Opinions are divided regarding the necessity of such distribution-free tests. Their use is strongly supported by some workers, whilst others believe that in a large majority of cases the parametric tests are sufficiently 'robust' to make them unnecessary. In other words, even if any assumption concerning the distribution is not fully justified, the tests are not unduly affected. These tests are, however, widely used and it is important to gain some familiarity with them.

The Mann–Whitney or Wilcoxon rank-sum test

This test is the non-parametric equivalent of the independent or two-sample t-test. It is based on a test that was originally devised by Wilcoxon and developed by Mann and Whitney, and may be encountered in two slightly different forms. Care should be taken not to confuse this test with the Wilcoxon signed-ranks test, which is considered later in this chapter, and for that reason it is perhaps best referred to as the Mann–Whitney test.

The form illustrated in this chapter, which is the approach most commonly encountered, considers a quantity known as the Mann–Whitney statistic U, the nature of which is explained in the example which follows. The Wilcoxon rank-sum test described in some texts employs the rank-sum directly, whereby the corresponding tables are, of course, rather different, but the final conclusion will be the same. That approach, it could be argued, is rather more straightforward, but it is less common, and for this reason is not considered here.

The principle of the Mann–Whitney test

If both samples are the same size and the mean of each is the same, we would expect, if the two sets of data were combined and ranked, that the sums of the ranks for each sample would be the same, or nearly so. Since they are not necessarily the same size, the difference between the observed sum of the ranks and the minimum possible sum of the ranks is calculated and this is referred to as the Mann–Whitney statistic, U.

The minimum possible sum of the ranks

In the following example, if all the data in both groups are combined and ranked, the sum of the ranks for group A would be a minimum if all the values in that sample were smaller than the values in group B, i.e. the ranks were 1, 2, 3, 4 and 5, the sum of which is given by $(4 \times 5)/2$. In general, this sum is given by $n(n + 1)/2$, where n is the size of the sample.

Example 9.1

Consider two samples which represent the number of visits to an osteopath required to obtain relief from a particular type of lower back problem when two different kinds of treatment were employed.

Five patients were given treatment A, and six were given B:

	Number of sessions					
Treatment A	7	9	10	5	9	
Treatment B	5	4	8	4	7	5

Can it be concluded that the two treatments are equally effective?

Firstly, the data from both samples are combined and ranked:

No of sessions	Treatment	Rank
4	B	1.5
4	B	1.5
5	B	4
5	B	4
5	A	4
7	A	6.5
7	B	6.5
8	B	8
9	A	9.5
9	A	9.5
10	A	11

With small samples such as we have in this example, this does not present much of a problem. With larger samples, however, if this is to be done by hand, the easiest approach is firstly to scan the data and estimate the smallest and largest items, whereupon a crude scale, covering this range, can then be set up on the left-hand side of a clean sheet of paper so that each data item can be placed in the appropriate position in the scale and the sample to which it belongs may be added in brackets. It is then a relatively simple task to write a list of data ranked in order of magnitude.

The hypotheses

A mentioned above, the Mann–Whitney test is the non-parametric equivalent of the independent sample *t*-test. However, unlike the *t*-test, no assumptions are made regarding the nature of the distributions and the null hypothesis is generally stated in a rather less specific form which simply asserts that the two samples come from identical populations, rather than from populations with the same mean. The alternative hypotheses are, for a two-way test, that the populations are not identical, and for a one-way test, that the values in one population are, in general, larger (or smaller) than in the other.

The treatment of tied ranks

Note that in the case of tied ranks an average value is assigned to each, i.e. the two values of 4 are ranked 1.5 each, rather than 1 and 2, and the three values of 5 are ranked 4, rather than 3, 4 and 5. This is, of course, not strictly necessary if the tied ranks are in the same sample but may be done for the sake of consistency. The sums of the ranks for each group, which may be arbitrarily designated W_1 and W_2, are then obtained:

$$W_1 = 4 + 6.5 + 9.5 + 9.5 + 11 \quad = 40.5$$
$$W_2 = 1.5 + 1.5 + 4 + 4 + 6.5 + 8 = 25.5$$

Calculation of the Mann–Whitney U statistic

The U statistic is a measure of the difference between the observed sum of the ranks for a sample and the minimum possible sum of the ranks. Thus the smaller is the value of U, the closer is the observed rank sum to the minimum, which would be observed if *all* the observations in the sample being considered were less than those in the second sample and, hence, the less likely it is that the null hypothesis is true.

U may now be calculated for each sample:

$$U_1 = W_1 - \frac{n_1(n_1 + 1)}{2} = 40.5 - \frac{5(6)}{2} = 25.5$$

$$U_2 = W_2 - \frac{n_2(n_2 + 1)}{2} = 25.5 - \frac{6(7)}{2} = 4.5$$

$$(9.1)$$

The significance of U

For a two-way, or non-directional test, U, the smaller value of U_1 or U_2, is compared with the tabulated value. The smaller is the value of U, the less likely is it that it has occurred by chance if the null hypothesis is true. Thus the null hypothesis is rejected in favour of the alternative if the observed value of U is less than, or equal to, the tabulated value for the appropriate sample sizes and significance level.

We can see that U_1 will be small when W_1 is small, and U_2 will be small when W_2 is small, thus for a one-way test, it is also the smaller value which is compared with the tabulated value, although the significance for a given value of U is half that for the two-way test.

Thus, if we test the null hypothesis against the alternative that the two populations are not identical, i.e. a two-way test, we find, from Table E in Appendix VI, that with $n_1 = 5$ and $n_2 = 6$ at the 5% level of significance $(P = 0.05)$, the critical value of U is 3.

From Equation 9.1 we see that the observed value of U_2 is less than U_1 and is equal to 4.5, thus:

$$U_{\text{observed}} > U_{\text{Critical}}$$

so that the null hypothesis cannot be rejected. We would therefore conclude that there is not a significant difference between the two types of treatment at the 5% level.

An approximation to the normal distribution

The tables that are available for the interpretation of the Mann–Whitney U statistic are generally limited to relatively small samples. If either, or both, of the samples is larger than about 20, advantage may be taken of the fact that, as the samples become large, the distribution of the U statistic approaches, and may be approximated to, the normal distribution. The mean and standard deviation of which are given by:

$$\mu_U = \frac{n_1 n_2}{2}$$

$$\sigma_U = \sqrt{\frac{n_1 n_2 (n_1 + n_2 + 1)}{12}}$$

(9.2)

Calculation of Z

Since the mean and standard deviation may be determined, Z may be calculated using either value of U. U_1 and U_2 will be symmetrically astride the mean value $(n_1 n_2/2)$, thus the smaller and larger values will give the left and right tail probabilities respectively.

$$Z = \frac{U - \mu_U}{\sigma_U} \qquad (9.3)$$

The significance may be determined from the normal distribution tables. This is illustrated in the following example.

Example 9.2

Consider the following two samples of sizes 20 and 22 respectively.

Sample 1	31	28	24	31	24	24	28	23	25	28
	31	32	31	29	22	30	30	22	28	24

Sample 2	28	22	31	24	20	28	22	22	23	24
	31	22	27	26	22	25	25	28	22	29
	24	25								

If the data are ranked, the following values are obtained for the two samples:

$$n_1 = 20 \qquad\qquad n_2 = 22$$
$$W_1 = 511.5 \qquad\qquad W_2 = 391.5$$
$$\frac{n_1(n_1 + 1)}{2} = 210 \qquad\qquad \frac{n_2(n_2 + 1)}{2} = 253$$
$$U_1 = 511.5 - 210 \qquad\qquad U_2 = 391.5 - 253$$
$$= 301.5 \qquad\qquad = 138.5$$

The mean and standard deviation of the U statistic are:

$$\mu_U = \frac{n_1 n_2}{2} \qquad \sigma_U = \sqrt{\frac{n_1 n_2(n_1 + n_2 + 1)}{12}}$$
$$= \frac{(20)(22)}{2} \qquad = \sqrt{\frac{(20)(22)(43)}{12}}$$
$$= 220 \qquad = 39.71$$

so that:

$$Z = \frac{301.5 - 220}{39.71} \quad \text{or} \quad Z = \frac{138.5 - 220}{39.71}$$

$$= +2.05 \qquad\qquad = -2.05$$

The significance of Z

Reference to the normal distribution tables shows that, if the null hypothesis is true, the probability that Z will be less than 2.05 is 0.9798, i.e. the probability that it will exceed this value is $(1 - 0.9798) = 0.0202$. Since the distribution is symmetrical about $Z = 0$, the probability that it will be less than -2.05 is also 0.0202. Thus, for a two-way test, $P = 0.0404$, or for a one-way test, $P = 0.0202$.

A two-way test

If we are testing the null hypothesis against the alternative that the two populations are not the same, that is a two-way test, the probability that the observed result has occurred by chance is only 0.0404, or 4.04%. If we are working at the 5% level of significance, this means that the null hypothesis would be rejected in favour of the alternative and we would conclude that the two populations are different, or that the difference 'is significant at the 5% level' or

$$P = 0.04$$

A one-way test

If, however, the alternative hypothesis is that the data in Sample 1 are greater than in Sample 2, i.e. a one-way or directional test, then the difference 'is significant at the 2.5% level' or

$$P = 0.02$$

In these cases, we can quote a specific value for P because we are referring to the normal distribution tables.

The Wilcoxon matched-pairs signed-ranks test

This test is the non-parametric equivalent of the paired-sample (related) t-test and, as in the case of the Mann–Whitney test considered above, no assumptions are made regarding the nature of the distribution so the null and alternative hypotheses are the same as in the above test.

Remember that, as with the paired sample t-test, each observation must have an identifiable partner.

This test also gives us a non-parametric equivalent to the one-sample t-test, where the differences between each value in the sample and a specified population mean are considered. This is just like a paired sample test except one of the pairs has a constant value, the specified population mean.

Principle of the test

The numerical values of the differences between each pair of observations, *without* regard to the sign, are ranked. Any differences which are zero, i.e. the value in each sample is identical, are ignored, and an average rank is allocated to those which are equal in the same way as in the Mann–Whitney test. Although the differences are ranked without regard to sign, it is necessary to record which are positive and which are negative and the sum of the ranks of each of these is calculated and given the symbol W_+ and W_- respectively.

If the null hypothesis is true, we would expect that W_+ and W_- would be approximately equal. If the null hypothesis is not true, one of them will be small and the other large. The smaller of the two is given the symbol W and is compared with the percentage points of the signed rank distribution, Table F in Appendix VI.

Example 9.3

An experiment was conducted to determine whether a patient's perception of the quality of treatment in a hospital clinic differed significantly from that in a private practice. Eight volunteers were asked to visit two physiotherapists, one in a hospital clinic and the second in private practice. They were then asked to indicate on a ten-point scale whether they felt that the treatment was beneficial with the following results:

	A	B	C	D	E	F	G	H
NHS	7	5	7	8	6	8	7	8
Private	7	7	8	6	9	4	4	4

Since each patient visited both locations, this represents a 'repeated measures' test, and since we may feel uncertain regarding the nature of the distribution of the responses, a non-parametric test is preferred. Therefore we shall apply a Wilcoxon matched-pairs or signed-ranks test, which is the non-parametric equivalent of the paired sample t-test.

The differences are ranked, *ignoring the sign* and excluding any differences of zero. As before, tied ranks are given an average value. The sums of the ranks of the positive and negative differences (W_+ and W_- respectively) are then calculated.

The scores allocated by each patient together with the differences and ranks of the differences are shown in the following table:

Patient	Treatment in clinic	Private treatment	Difference in score	Rank of difference ignoring the sign
A	7	7	0	–
B	5	7	-2	2.5 $(-)$
C	7	8	-1	1 $(-)$
D	8	6	2	2.5 $(+)$
E	6	9	-3	4.5 $(-)$
F	8	4	4	6.5 $(+)$
G	7	4	3	4.5 $(+)$
H	8	4	4	6.5 $(+)$

From the above it can be seen that:

$$W_+ = 2.5 + 6.5 + 4.5 + 6.5 \quad = 20$$
$$W_- = 2.5 + 1 + 4.5 \quad\quad\quad = 8$$

The significance of W

The smaller of the two values, $W_- = 8$, is taken to be W and is compared with the critical values given in Table F. To be significant, the observed value must be equal to, or less than, the appropriate critical value. Remember that if the sum of the ranks of one particular sign is large, the sum for the opposite sign will be small, and the smaller it becomes, the less likely it is that it has occurred by chance and that the null hypothesis is true. If this hypothesis is true, i.e. that the average difference between the ranks is zero, we expect the sums to be about equal.

For a test of the null hypothesis against a two-sided alternative, that the treatments are different, the critical value for $n = 7$ (the zero difference is not counted) at the 5% level of significance ($P = 0.05$) is found to be 2. In the above example, W is considerably larger than 2, so the null hypothesis cannot be rejected and it would be concluded that there is not a significant difference between the patients' perceptions of the efficacy of the treatment in the two locations.

For a one-tailed test, where the experimental or alternative hypothesis is that one specified treatment is better than the other, once again the smaller value of W is compared with the critical value. In this case, of course, the significance level is one half that for the two-way test.

An approximation to the normal distribution

As with the Mann–Whitney test considered earlier, an approximation to the normal distribution is possible when n becomes large, generally taken to be greater than 15. In this case the sum of the ranks approximately follows a normal distribution with mean and standard deviation given by:

$$\mu_w = \frac{n(n+1)}{4}$$

$$\sigma_w = \sqrt{\frac{n(n+1)(2n+1)}{24}}$$

(9.4)

so that, as before Z may be calculated and the significance determined from the normal distribution tables.

Kruskal–Wallis test

This test is a non-parametric equivalent of the one-way ANOVA and, as such, is an extension of the Mann–Whitney U test for more than two samples, i.e. it is used to compare the means of more than two samples when the data are ordinal. The null hypothesis is that all samples are drawn from identical populations.

The procedure is as follows. The data are all combined together and ranked, but a record is kept of the ranks for each group. The sums of the ranks of the members of each group are computed. These are denoted by R_A, R_B, etc., which, if the null hypothesis is true, we would expect to be more or less equal if we make allowance for differences in sample size. The statistic H is a measure of the degree to which the sums of the ranks differ from one another:

$$H = \frac{12}{N(N+1)} \sum \frac{R^2}{n} - 3(N+1)$$

(9.5)

where:

$R =$ the sum of a particular group,
$n =$ the number of observations in that group,
$k =$ the number of groups (samples),
$N =$ the total number of observations $(\sum n)$.

Provided all the samples contain at least five observations, the distribution of H approximates to the χ^2 and its value may be compared for significance against the critical values of χ^2 (Table C) at $(k-1)$ degrees of freedom. For smaller samples, much more extensive tables are required such as those given in the *New Cambridge Elementary Statistical Tables.*

The way in which H is calculated is shown in the following example.

Example 9.4

24 therapists, divided at random into three groups, attended computer usage courses at three different institutions. On completion of the course, they were asked to take an assessment and the following marks were achieved.

Group A	Group B	Group C
63	72	50
55	85	58
65	75	35
82	80	55
80	45	40
76	60	50
54	67	39
65	56	42

We shall use a Kruskal–Wallis test to determine if the results from the three courses are significantly different.

All the data are sorted in order and ranked. As before, tied values are given an average rank:

Rank	Data	Group	
1	35		C
2	39		C
3	40		C
4	42		C
5	45	B	
6.5	50		C
6.5	50		C
8	54	A	

continued

continued

Rank	Data	Group		
9.5	55	A		
9.5	55			C
11	56		B	
12	58			C
13	60		B	
14	63	A		
15.5	65	A		
15.5	65	A		
17	67		B	
18	72		B	
19	75		B	
20	76	A		
21.5	80	A		
21.5	80		B	
23	82	A		
24	85		B	

From which we can determine the sum of the ranks for each group:

$$R_A = 8 + 9.5 + 14 + 15.5 + 15.5 + 20 + 21.5 + 23 = 127$$
$$R_B = 5 + 11 + 13 + 17 + 18 + 19 + 21.5 + 24 = 128.5$$
$$R_C = 1 + 2 + 3 + 4 + 6.5 + 6.5 + 9.5 + 12 = 44.5$$

The statistic H may now be calculated using Equation 9.5:

$$H = \frac{12}{24(24 + 1)}\left[\frac{127^2}{8} + \frac{128.5^2}{8} + \frac{44.5^2}{8}\right] - 3(24 + 1)$$
$$= 11.55$$

From the tables giving the critical values of χ^2 we find that, at 2 degrees of freedom:

$$\chi^2_{0.005} = 10.60$$

which means that if the null hypothesis (that the three populations are identical) is true, there is a probability of 0.005 or 0.5% that χ^2 will take a value as large as, or larger than, 10.60 by chance. Thus a value of 11.55 will occur by chance with a probability less than this, i.e.

$$P < 0.005$$

The probability that the observed value will occur, even if the null hypothesis is true, is only 0.5% or less. This represents the risk, which is very small, of being wrong if we reject it. Thus the probability that we are right is 99.5%, so it may be said that we reject with 99.5% confidence and conclude that there is a significant difference in at least one of the populations.

In common with the ANOVA, the Kruskal–Wallis test will simply tell us that there is a difference and no more, i.e. it is a non-directional or two-way test. However, in this case if we look at the sums of the ranks, we see that the sum for Group C is very much less than that for A or B, which are very close to each other, and since a low rank corresponds to a low score, we would be justified in concluding that the scores in Group C are, in general, less than in either of the other two groups.

The Friedman test

The Friedman test is the non-parametric equivalent of the two-way ANOVA, or the one-way with repeated measures which, you will remember, is the extension of the paired sample, or related t-test (a parametric test) to more than two samples. As in the other non-parametric tests, the Friedman test makes no assumptions about the nature of the distributions involved.

In this test the scores *for each subject* under each condition are ranked, thus if there are three conditions, the rankings for each subject will be 1, 2 and 3, although, of course, not necessarily in that order. The appropriate statistic is given the symbol M and is computed:

$$M = \frac{12}{nk(k+1)} \sum R^2 - 3n(k+1) \qquad (9.6)$$

where:
  R = the sum of the ranks for a given condition or group,
  n = the number of subjects (patients),
  k = the number of conditions (repeated measures).

The critical values of Friedman statistic M are given in Table J in Appendix VI. For large samples the distribution of this statistic tends to the χ^2 distribution (Table C) at $(k - 1)$ degrees of freedom.

Example 9.5

In an evaluation of reliability, a particular test was applied to six stroke patients on three successive days by different assessors. The test involved rather subjective assessments to give a maximum score of 25. The following results were obtained:

Patient	Day 1 Score	Day 1 Rank	Day 2 Score	Day 2 Rank	Day 3 Score	Day 3 Rank
A	12	1	14	2	18	3
B	9	1	20	2	23	3
C	10	2	8	1	17	3
D	6	1	8	2	11	3
E	16	3	9	1	13	2
F	11	2	10	1	16	3
Rank sum $(R) =$	10		9		17	

Note that the scores have been ranked for each subject, i.e. across the rows. Can it be concluded that the three assessments are not significantly different from each other?

From the data:

$$M = \frac{12}{(6)(3)(3 + 1)}(10^2 + 9^2 + 17^2) - (3)(6)(3 + 1)$$
$$= 6.33$$

Since there are six patients measured under three different conditions, $n = 6$ and $k = 3$. Reference to Table J shows that:

$$M_{0.10} = 5.33$$
$$M_{0.05} = 7.00$$

Our calculated value of 6.33 lies between these two, thus we would conclude that:

$$0.05 < P < 0.10$$

i.e. there is more than a 5% probability that the differences have occurred by chance, so we would accept the null hypothesis and conclude that the three assessors do agree with each other.

It is worth noting that if there is not a significant difference between the three assessments we would expect the sum of the ranks under each condition to be (more or less) the same, which in Example 9.5 would be 12 in each case, whereupon the value of M is zero. Remember that as n becomes large, the distribution of M tends to that of χ^2 and thus the larger its value, the lower is the probability that it has arisen by chance and conversely, of course, the smaller it is, the greater is the probability that it has arisen by chance.

Summary

THE MANN–WHITNEY RANK-SUM TEST is a non-parametric equivalent to the two-sample t-test and is used to compare the means of two samples when they cannot be assumed to follow, at least approximately, a normal distribution.
THE WILCOXON PAIRED-SAMPLE SIGNED-RANKS TEST is a non-parametric equivalent to the paired-sample or related t-test. It is used to compare two sets of data obtained by 'repeated measures', e.g. a 'before' and 'after' comparison, or a group of subjects where a measurement is taken for each subject under two different conditions. The crucial criterion is that any particular observation must have an identifiable partner. This test may also be used to compare a sample with a specified population mean.
THE KRUSKAL–WALLIS TEST is a non-parametric equivalent to the one-way ANOVA, that is to say it is an extension of the Mann–Whitney test on more than two samples.
THE FRIEDMAN TEST is the non-parametric equivalent of the one-way ANOVA with repeated measures and is thus an extension of the Wilcoxon paired-sample signed-ranks test on more than two samples.

Exercises for Chapter 9

Exercise 9.1

The following data represent a scale indicating a level of difficulty with speech in two groups of patients who suffer from Parkinson's disease. The patients in Group B have received an operation to treat the disease, the control Group A had no operation.

Is there a significant difference in the difficulty experienced by each group?

Group A	1.5	1.5	2.8	2.5	1.9	1.9	2.0	2.7	1.5
Group B	1.2	0.8	1.6	1.8	1.6	1.9	1.9		

Exercise 9.2

A study was undertaken to compare two methods of training patients in the use of a particular walking aid. It was claimed that Method I was superior to Method II. Two groups of patients were selected at random and the effectiveness of each method was measured by the time (in days) it took to achieve a certain standard.

The following data were collected.

Method I	3	7	2	4	2	5			
Method II	4	6	8	7	3	5	7	6	4

Is the claim justified? Work at a 5% level of significance.

Exercise 9.3

As a useful exercise to emphasize the importance of sample sizes, consider the data given in Exercise 9.2 and assume that the sample sizes are doubled by duplicating the data in each case. Perform a similar test and compare the result with that obtained in the above exercise. Clearly the mean, or median, and the variability must be the same in each circumstance, but quite a different result is obtained.

Note that, if you calculate the standard deviations for the data, for example, for method I in Exercise 9.2 and then after duplication as suggested in this exercise, the same result will be obtained only if the data are treated as populations because, in the case of a sample, the variance involves division by the number of degrees of freedom, i.e. $(n - 1)$, rather than by n, as in the case of a population. Thus if $n = 6$ and $n = 12$, as in Exercise 9.2 and this exercise, to obtain the variances the sums of the squares, which, of course will differ exactly by a factor of 2, are divided by 5 and 11, respectively.

Exercise 9.4

A cohort of 36 students was divided at random into three equal groups taking clinical placements in three different institutions. The assessments, on a ten-point scale, given by these institutions were as follows.

Group A	7	4	5	5	4	6	4	5	8	8	6	6
Group B	7	4	9	9	8	6	10	5	10	5	8	6
Group C	9	5	8	8	6	8	5	6	7	10	5	8

Use a Kruskal–Wallis test at a 5% significance level to test the hypothesis that there is no difference between the three groups of assessments.

Exercise 9.5

A group of ten patients who were about to undergo treatment involving traction were rated according to their anxiety levels. A five-point scale was used, 0 representing low anxiety and 5 representing high anxiety. The patients were then shown an explanatory video and rated again. The ratings were as follows:

Before viewing the video	2 2 3 0 3 1 1 3 1 0
After viewing the video	1 0 0 0 3 1 2 0 0 0

Test the hypothesis that showing the video reduces the anxiety of the patient.

Exercise 9.6

An experiment was conducted to compare three different approaches to the presentation of a training programme. Five tutors were asked to present the same programme to three different audiences using a different method each time, Method A using a lot of visual aids, Method B showing a videotape and Method C presenting the audience with printed notes. Each audience was asked to rate the presentation on a 20-point scale and the average value in each case was taken as the variable for comparison. The following scores were obtained:

Tutor	Method		
	A	B	C
1	15	10	17
2	12	11	19
3	17	13	17
4	14	10	15
5	10	12	11

Test the hypothesis that the three methods are equally effective against the alternative that they are not.

Glossary of Common Statistical Terms

Accuracy A measure of how close a determination is to the 'true value'. Usually, of course, this is not known and is, in fact, that which we are endeavouring to find. This should not be confused with precision.

Alternative hypothesis *See* experimental hypothesis.

Analysis of variance (ANOVA) A statistical test used to compare the means of more than two samples.

Barchart A chart used to display the frequency with which certain events have occurred.

Categorical data *See* nominal data.

Chi-square test A test used with nominal data to compare proportions, or as a test for independence.

Class mark The mid-point, or characteristic value, of a class or group in a histogram.

Coefficient of variation The standard deviation represented as a percentage of the mean which thus gives a better indication of the relative variability of the observations.

Confidence interval The range of values within which we have a specified confidence that the population parameter which we have estimated will be found.

Confidence level   The degree of confidence, expressed as a percentage, that may be placed on an estimate of a population parameter. The most common level is 95%.

Contingency table   A table showing observed and expected frequencies used in the chi-square test.

Continuous data   Data which result from measurements, where the precision with which it is measured is dependent only on the instrument used for that purpose.

Correlation coefficient   A measure of the strength of a linear relationship between pairs of observations. It is defined in such a way that it may take values only between -1.0 and $+1.0$, and the closer it is to these values, the stronger is the negative or positive association respectively.

Critical value   The value of a statistic which, as the result of theoretical arguments, is likely to occur by chance with a specified probability. For example, ina t-test, the value of t which would occur by chance with, say, a probability of 0.05 or 5%, so that, if the observed value exceeds this critical value, the probability that it has occurred by chance is less than 5% so we would conclude that the result is 'significant' at the 5% level.

Cumulative density function (CDF)   A measure of the cumulative probability density below a specific value of a statistic, i.e. the probability that a value less than the specified value will be observed.

Cumulative frequency plot   The cumulative frequency is the number, often represented as a percentage, of observations below the upper boundary of each particular class in a histogram. Thus, for any particular value of the random variable (the observed or measured quantity) the plot gives the percentage of observations falling below that value.

Degrees of freedom   The number of values in a set of data which may be changed without altering the overall nature of the set. In the simplest case, for a set of n observations, $(n - 1)$ may be freely changed but the last observation must have a specific value if the mean, or sum total, is to remain unaltered. Thus we have $(n - 1)$ degrees of freedom, usually abbreviated to df, although other symbols may well be encountered, e.g. ν ('nu') or, perhaps, ϕ ('phi').

Dependent variable   In general, this is the quantity which is measured. Its value depends upon the manipulation of the 'independent variable', which is the one controlled by the observer.

Descriptive statistics   Techniques which are concerned with describing data, for example, using graphs, pie charts, bar charts or histograms. Such methods of display give an instant visual impression so that information may be assimilated more readily. It is very difficult to gain a general impression from a page full of numbers.

Determinate errors   Errors, the cause of which may, at least in principle, be identified and thereby corrected, e.g. using wrongly calibrated equipment.

Discrete data   Data which exist only in the form of whole numbers, for example, when events or objects are counted.

Experimental hypothesis   Usually given the symbol H_1, it is an alternative to the null hypothesis, H_0 (which asserts that there is no difference between two variables being compared) and asserts that the latter is not true and that a true difference exists.

Frequency distribution   A histogram which displays the frequency with which the values within a particular group or class are observed.

Friedman test   A non-parametric test for comparing populations involving repeated measures under different conditions for a single group of subjects. Equivalent to the parametric one-way ANOVA with repeated measures, or two-way ANOVA.

F-test   A statistical test used to compare two variances.

Gross error   *See* determinate error.

Histogram   A form of barchart where continuous data are fitted into a number of 'classes' or 'groups', and the frequency of occurrence within each group is displayed. The general nature of the distribution can be seen more readily.

Independent variable   The variable which is under the control of the experimenter and is manipulated in order that the effect on the 'dependent variable' may be observed.

Indeterminate error   *See* random variation or error.

Inferential statistics   Techniques which are concerned with drawing inferences about a population from data collected from a sample.

Interquartile range   The range which excludes the lowest quarter and the highest quarter of a set of data and thus includes the middle 50% of the observations.

Interval data   Data measured on a uniform scale, but with an arbitrary zero, e.g. the Celsius scale of temperature.

Kendall's coefficient of concordance   A non-parametric statistical test which assesses the general agreement between more than two sets of data.

Kruskal–Wallis test   A non-parametric test for comparing more than two populations. Equivalent to the parametric one-way ANOVA.

Level of significance   *See* significance level.

Linear regression   A statistical technique whereby an equation is obtained giving the most probable value of the dependent variable (y) as a function of the independent variable (x). This 'regression equation' may be used to estimate values of y for any given value of x, or may be used to draw 'the line of best fit' through a scatterplot of the points on a graph. Sometimes referred to as the method of least squares.

Mann–Whitney U test   Equivalent to the Wilcoxon rank-sum test. A non-parametric equivalent to the independent sample t-test.

Mean   In everyday language, this is the average, i.e. all measurements are added and the total is divided by the number of measurements taken. This is the most common measure of central tendency and is given the symbol $\bar{x}$ or μ when representing a sample or population respectively. Remember that $\bar{x}$ is a statistic and μ is a parameter.

Measures of central tendency   Such a measure is simply a 'characteristic' number representing a set of data (measurements or observations), e.g. the mean or the median.

Median   The middle value of a set of data, or that value below which 50% of the observations are to be found when they are sorted into numerical order. If there is an odd number of observations, there is a distinct middle value, if an even number, then the average of the two middle values is taken.

Method of least squares   *See* linear regression.

Mode   The mode, as the name suggests, represents the most 'fashionable' or common value. It is, however, usually reserved for 'nominal' or 'categorical' data which may be represented on a bar chart, and thus indicates the most common category.

Nominal data   Sometimes referred to as categorical data, where observations are place into categories.

Non-parametric test   A test which does not rely on estimation of population parameters and makes no assumptions regarding the nature of the distribution.

Normal distribution   A bell-shaped distribution curve which represents many sets of data which are subject to random effects. It is the most fundamental of all frequency distributions and is crucial to the concept of statistical inference.

Null hypothesis   Given the symbol H_0, this hypothesis asserts that there is no difference (hence 'null') between the variables being compared. It is accepted, by defult, if insufficient evidence is found to support the experimental or alternative hypothesis.

One-way test   Alternatively referred to as a one-tailed or directional test. A statistical test in which the experimental hypothesis asserts that the mean of a particular sample is larger, or perhaps smaller, than the sample with which it is being compared, rather than simply different.

Ordinal data   Data which can be replaced in rank order but cannot be considered to be on a scale of measurement.

Parameter   A property of a population, e.g. the mean or standard deviation. This has a fixed value, because the composition of the population is fixed. It is, however, usually unknown and is the quantity that we are endeavouring to determine and is estimated by a sample statistic.

Parametric test   A test for which the data must be interval or ratio and the assumption is made that the sampling distribution is, at least approximately, normal, e.g. the t-test.

Pearson product moment correlation coefficient   *See* correlation coefficient.

Pooled estimate of variance or standard deviation   An estimate of the variance or standard deviation for the population based on the assumption that the values calculated for several samples are not significantly different from each other and are thus independent estimates of the same population value. The value so obtained is 'weighted' according to the number of degrees of freedom in each sample.

Population   This term, used to indicate the total possible number of observations, has persisted because of the fact that the subject of statistics was originally concerned with estimating requirements of, or information about, whole populations from a section of that population. It now has a more general meaning and represents the total possible number of observations.

Precision   A measurement of the reproducibility of measurements. The smaller the standard deviation, the more precise is a set of measurements. This should not be confused with accuracy.

Probability density function (PDF)   The height of the probability curve for any given value of an observation or statistic.

P-value   The probability that an observed effect is simply the result of random variation.

Random sample   *See* sample.

Random variable   The name given to the observed quantity implying that it varies as a result of random factors.

Random variation or error   The variability in a set of data that occurs naturally or over which we have no control. In the case of measurements, it is sometimes referred to as indeterminate error, because it results from random factors which cannot be eliminated, although with care can be reduced. Variance and standard deviation are measures of random variation.

Ratio scale   A scale with a true zero, e.g. weight or length.

Regression equation   The equation which describes the line of best fit through a series of points in a graph.

Repeated measures   A test where a dependent variable is measured several times for each subject under different conditions, e.g. a paired sample *t*-test or ANOVA.

Residuals   The differences between the observed and the fitted values obtained by regression analysis.

Sample   That section ('subset') of the population on which we make our measurements or observations so that we may make inferences about the population, such as an estimation of the mean. It should be selected at random, that is, every member of the population should have an equal chance of being included.

Scatterplot   A term used to describe a plot in which points corresponding to particular pairs of observations are plotted on *x*–*y* axes.

Significance level   Commonly set at 5%, although other levels may be used if appropriate. A result is said to be 'significant at the 5% level' if the probability that it has occurred by chance is less than 5%, i.e. there is only a small probability that it *has* occurred by chance, so we conclude that a real difference exists between the parameters being compared. We should remember, of course, that this means there is (at most) a 5% chance that we are wrong.

Skewed   This term refers to a frequency distribution which is asymmetrical.

Spearman rank correlation coefficient   A non-parametric correlation coefficient for ranked data.

Standard deviation   The square root of the variance. A measure of variability which is rather more convenient than the more fundamental variance because it has the same dimensions as the mean.

Standard error of the mean   The standard deviation of the means of a large number of samples taken from the same population.

Standard normal distribution   The normal distribution with zero mean and unit standard deviation.

Statistic   A property of a sample, e.g. the mean or standard deviation. This does not have a fixed value because it will vary from one sample to another as a result of random effects. Each sample statistic is an independent estimate of the corresponding population parameter.

t-test   A *t*-test is used in the comparison of means. In general there are three kinds.

—A one-sample test to compare the mean of the population from which a sample was taken with a specified population mean.

—An independent sample test to compare the means of two independent samples.

—A related or paired-sample test for repeated measures, e.g. a 'before' and 'after' test with difference subjects.

Two-way test   Alternatively referred to as a two tailed or non-directional test. A statistical test in which the experimental or alternative hypothesis does not specify the direction in which a difference between the parameters under test exists, simply that they are different.

Variance   A measure of the variability of a set of data. Sometimes referred to as 'the mean sum of the squares', which may be a little confusing, because, strictly, it is 'the mean sum of the squares of the differences between each observation and the mean'.

Wilcoxon rank-sum test   Equivalent to the Mann–Whitney test except the sum of the ranks is tabulated instead of the U statistic. A non-parametric equivalent of the independent sample t-test.

Wilcoxon signed-ranks test   The non-parametric equivalent of the paired sample t-test.

Yates continuity correction   A correction applied when conducting a chi-square test with a 2×2 contingency table when there is only a single degree of freedom.

II

Significant Figures, Decimal Places and Scientific Notation

Significant Figures and Decimal Places

The number of significant figures and the number of decimal places are often confused. The former is an indication of the precision that can be expected of a measurement, whilst the latter may simply be a measure of the 'order of magnitude' or size of a number.

For example, it is tempting to believe that a number such as 0.000 03 is measured with a high degree of precision (remember that precision is a measure of reproducibility). This number is represented to five decimal places, i.e. there are five digits after the decimal point. It is, nevertheless, not very precise, because the implication is that the measurement is 'somewhere between' 0.000 025 and 0.000 035. It is thus given to only a single significant figure. If, however, it had been represented as 0.000 030, which implies a value between 0.000 029 5 and 0.000 030 5, this is clearly rather more precise and is represented to two significant figures.

Similarly, 0.000 030 0 is represented to three significant figures, and, of course, to seven decimal places. Thus it is clear that the number of decimal places and the number of significant figures do not necessarily have any relation.

Scientific notation

A difficulty arises with very large and very small numbers, for example, it might be said that 50,000 people attend a rally. No one would take that to mean *exactly* 50,000, but it is not possible, from that number, to assess how close the exact number is to 50,000. On the other hand, if it had been said that 50,324 people were present, we would accept that as an exact count. That is, in the latter case, the number is represented to give five significant figures, but, in the former, it is not possible to draw a conclusion about the number of significant figures.

If, however, the number is represented in scientific notation, e.g. 5×10^4 (i.e. $5 \times 10 \times 10 \times 10 \times 10$), the number of significant figures may clearly be seen, e.g. 5×10^4, 5.0×10^4, 5.00×10^4, and so on, indicating one, two and three significant figures respectively. Thus if the count was exactly 50,000, it could be represented as 5.0000×10^4. In a similar way, of course, 50,324 could be written as 5.0324×10^4.

Such a representation is clearly very useful when considering very large numbers, e.g. the number of molecules in 1.0 gram of water is about 33,500,000,000,000,000,000,000, which is a very cumbersome number. This may be written in the much more convenient form, 3.35×10^{22}.

Exactly the same procedure may be applied to very small numbers, e.g. the previous example, 0.000 03 may be written 3×10^{-5}, indicating one significant figure. If the measurement is more precise than that, it may be written 3.0×10^{-5}, 3.00×10^{-5}, and so on, for two or three significant figures respectively. Note that it is customary to quote the number multiplied by various powers of 10, with a single digit to the left of the decimal point.

Appendix
III

Statistical Formulae

Population standard deviation.

$$\sigma = \sqrt{\frac{1}{N}\sum(x - \mu)^2} = \sqrt{\frac{1}{N}\sum x^2 - N\mu^2}$$

Sample standard deviation.

$$s = \sqrt{\frac{1}{n-1}\sum(x - \bar{x})^2} = \sqrt{\frac{1}{n-1}\sum x^2 - n\bar{x}^2}$$

Z-statistic.

$$Z = \frac{x - \mu}{\sigma} \quad \text{or} \quad \frac{x - \mu_0}{\sigma/\sqrt{n}}$$

One-sample t-test.

A t-statistic to compare a sample mean with a specified population mean

$$t = \frac{\bar{x} - \mu_0}{s/\sqrt{n}}$$

Independent sample t-test.

A t-statistic to compare the means of two samples with $(n_A - 1) + (n_B - 1)$ degrees of freedom. Usually d_0 is zero:

$$t = \frac{(\bar{x}_A - \bar{x}_B) - d_0}{s_P \sqrt{\dfrac{1}{n_A} + \dfrac{1}{n_B}}}$$

where $s_P^2 =$ the pooled estimate of the variance:

$$s_P^2 = \frac{(n_A - 1)s_A^2 + (n_B - 1)s_B^2}{(n_A - 1) + (n_B - 1)} \quad \text{i.e. } s_P = \sqrt{s_P^2}$$

Paired sample (related) t-test.

A t-statistic when repeated measures are taken, $\bar{d}$ is the mean difference, s_d the standard deviation of the differences and μ_d is usually zero:

$$t = \frac{\bar{d} - \mu_d}{s_d / \sqrt{n}}$$

Chi-square statistic.

This compares proportions; a test for independence.

$$\chi^2 = \sum \frac{(O - E)^2}{E}$$

Pearson (product moment) correlation coefficient.

$$r = \frac{1}{(n - 1)} \frac{\sum xy - n\bar{x}\bar{y}}{s_x s_y}$$

Linear regression.

$$y = A + Bx \quad \text{where } B = \frac{\sum xy - n\bar{x}\bar{y}}{\sum x^2 - n\bar{x}^2} \text{ and } A = \bar{y} - B\bar{x}$$

Significance of the correlation coefficient using the t-statistic.

$$t = r\sqrt{\left(\frac{(n-2)}{(1-r^2)}\right)}$$

with $(n-2)$ degrees of freedom.

Analysis of variance (ANOVA)—one way.

The total 'sum of the squares' (SST) and the 'sum of the squares of the columns' (SSC) are required:

$$\text{SST} = \sum x^2 - \frac{G^2}{N} \quad df = (N-1)$$

$$\text{SSC} = \sum \frac{T^2}{n} - \frac{G^2}{N} \quad df = (k-1)$$

Analysis of variance (ANOVA)—two way or one-way with repeated measures.

In addition to the SST, the sums of the squares for the columns (SSC) and rows (SSR) are required:

$$\text{SSC} = \sum \frac{T_k^2}{n_r} - \frac{G^2}{N} \quad df = (k-1)$$

$$\text{SSR} = \sum \frac{T_r^2}{n_k} - \frac{G^2}{N} \quad df = (r-1)$$

Appendix

IV

The Correlation Coefficient

The correlation coefficient is defined as follows:

$$r = \frac{1}{n-1} \sum \frac{(x - \bar{x})(y - \bar{y})}{s_x s_y}$$

The following explanation may help you to appreciate the nature of the correlation coefficient and the reason for the definition being in this form.

The covariance of two sets of data is defined:

$$\text{Cov}(x, y) = \frac{1}{n-1} \sum (x - \bar{x})(y - \bar{y})$$

This definition is similar to that of the variance given in Chapter 2, except that $\sum (x - \bar{x})^2$ has been replaced by $\sum (x - \bar{x})(y - \bar{y})$.

If we look at the latter quantity we can see that if y is small when x is small, then both of these quantities will be less than their respective means, i.e. $(x - \bar{x})$ and $(y - \bar{y})$ will both be negative, and the product will thus be positive. If the value of y becomes large as x becomes large, then y will exceed $\bar{y}$ and x will exceed $\bar{x}$, thus $(y - \bar{y})$ and $(x - \bar{x})$ both become positive, and the product is, once more, positive. In this circumstance the covariance and the correlation coefficient will be positive. Thus if x and y both get larger together, the correlation coefficient is positive.

On the other hand, if y is large when x is small, $(y - \bar{y})$ will be positive when $(x - \bar{x})$ is negative, and if y becomes small as x becomes large, then $(y - \bar{y})$ and $(x - \bar{x})$ become negative and positive respectively, so that the product in each case is negative. In this case the covariance and correlation coefficient will be negative. Thus if y decreases as x increases, the correlation coefficient is negative.

It would be perfectly possible to accept the covariance as a measure of the extent of correlation (i.e. the strength of the relationship) between the two variables x and y, but its value would depend upon the particular values of x and y, and would be very difficult to interpret. For this reason it is 'standardized' by dividing the deviations from the mean of each variable by the standard deviations, i.e. $(x - \bar{x})/s_x$ and $(y - \bar{y})/s_y$. The result is the correlation coefficient defined above which may only take values between -1.0 and $+1.0$. Although it is defined in this way, the equation would not normally be used in this form to calculate the correlation coefficient (see Chapter 3, Equation 3.2).

Criteria for Test Selection

Decision tree for parametric tests

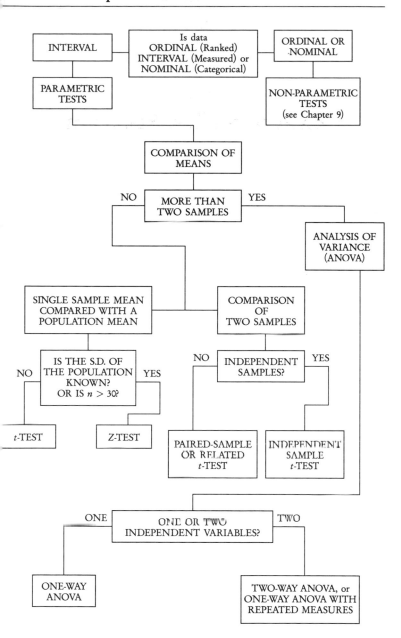

Non-parametric or distribution-free tests

Parametric tests are so called because they involve the estimation of parameters of the populations from which the samples are drawn. As a consequence, certain assumptions regarding the nature of those populations must therefore be made, namely that they follow, at least approximately, a normal distribution.

Although parametric tests are, in general, very 'robust', i.e. are relatively insensitive to deviations from these assumptions, if the sampling distributions deviate seriously from the normal, it is usually recommended that a non-parametric or distribution-free test is used.

Some statisticians believe that in the vast majority of cases, parametric tests are sufficiently robust to render the use of non-parametric tests unnecessary, whilst others are very strongly in favour of their use.

Decision tree for non-parametric tests

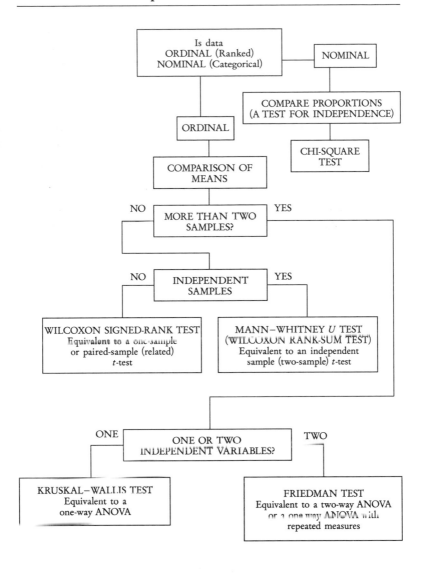

VI

Statistical Tables

Table A   The standard normal distribution

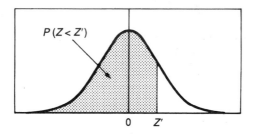

The table gives the area, $\phi(Z)$, shaded in the above diagram for any given positive value of Z, which represents the probability that Z will be *less* than that value. The probability that Z will be *more* than that value is $\{1 - \phi(Z)\}$.

Negative values of Z are not included because the distribution is symmetrical, thus the probability that Z will be less than a particular value Z' is the same as the probability that Z will exceed $-Z'$, i.e. $P(Z < Z') = P(Z > -Z')$.

The second decimal place for Z may be read by moving horizontally across the page.

Z	0.00	0.01	0.02	0.03	0.04	0.05	0.06	0.07	0.08	0.09
0.0	0.5000	0.5040	0.5080	0.5120	0.5160	0.5199	0.5239	0.5279	0.5319	0.5359
0.1	0.5398	0.5438	0.5478	0.5517	0.5557	0.5596	0.5636	0.5675	0.5714	0.5753
0.2	0.5793	0.5832	0.5871	0.5910	0.5948	0.5987	0.6026	0.6064	0.6103	0.6141
0.3	0.6179	0.6217	0.6255	0.6293	0.6331	0.6368	0.6406	0.6443	0.6480	0.6517
0.4	0.6554	0.6591	0.6628	0.6664	0.6700	0.6736	0.6772	0.6808	0.6844	0.6879
0.5	0.6915	0.6950	0.6985	0.7019	0.7054	0.7088	0.7123	0.7157	0.7190	0.7224
0.6	0.7257	0.7291	0.7324	0.7357	0.7389	0.7422	0.7454	0.7486	0.7517	0.7549
0.7	0.7580	0.7611	0.7642	0.7673	0.7704	0.7734	0.7764	0.7794	0.7823	0.7852
0.8	0.7881	0.7910	0.7939	0.7967	0.7995	0.8023	0.8051	0.8078	0.8106	0.8133
0.9	0.8159	0.8186	0.8212	0.8238	0.8264	0.8289	0.8315	0.8340	0.8365	0.8389
1.0	0.8413	0.8438	0.8461	0.8485	0.8508	0.8531	0.8554	0.8577	0.8599	0.8621
1.1	0.8643	0.8665	0.8686	0.8708	0.8729	0.8749	0.8770	0.8790	0.8810	0.8830
1.2	0.8849	0.8869	0.8888	0.8907	0.8925	0.8944	0.8962	0.8980	0.8997	0.9015
1.3	0.9032	0.9049	0.9066	0.9082	0.9099	0.9115	0.9131	0.9147	0.9162	0.9177
1.4	0.9192	0.9207	0.9222	0.9236	0.9251	0.9265	0.9279	0.9292	0.9306	0.9319
1.5	0.9332	0.9345	0.9357	0.9370	0.9382	0.9394	0.9406	0.9418	0.9429	0.9441
1.5	0.9452	0.9463	0.9474	0.9484	0.9495	0.9505	0.9515	0.9525	0.9535	0.9545
1.7	0.9554	0.9564	0.9573	0.9582	0.9591	0.9599	0.9608	0.9616	0.9625	0.9633
1.8	0.9641	0.9649	0.9656	0.9664	0.9671	0.9678	0.9686	0.9693	0.9699	0.9706
1.9	0.9713	0.9719	0.9726	0.9732	0.9738	0.9744	0.9750	0.9756	0.9761	0.9767
2.0	0.9772	0.9778	0.9783	0.9788	0.9793	0.9798	0.9803	0.9808	0.9812	0.9817
2.1	0.9821	0.9826	0.9830	0.9834	0.9838	0.9842	0.9846	0.9850	0.9854	0.9857
2.2	0.9861	0.9864	0.9868	0.9871	0.9875	0.9878	0.9881	0.9884	0.9887	0.9890
2.3	0.9893	0.9896	0.9898	0.9901	0.9904	0.9906	0.9909	0.9911	0.9913	0.9916
2.4	0.9918	0.9920	0.9922	0.9925	0.9927	0.9929	0.9931	0.9932	0.9934	0.9936
2.5	0.9938	0.9940	0.9941	0.9943	0.9945	0.9946	0.9948	0.9949	0.9951	0.9952
2.6	0.9953	0.9955	0.9956	0.9957	0.9959	0.9960	0.9961	0.9962	0.9963	0.9964
2.7	0.9965	0.9966	0.9967	0.9968	0.9969	0.9970	0.9971	0.9972	0.9973	0.9974
2.8	0.9974	0.9975	0.9976	0.9977	0.9977	0.9978	0.9979	0.9979	0.9980	0.9981
2.9	0.9981	0.9982	0.9982	0.9983	0.9984	0.9984	0.9985	0.9985	0.9986	0.9986
3.0	0.9986	0.9987	0.9987	0.9988	0.9988	0.9988	0.9989	0.9989	0.9990	0.9990

Table B   Critical values of the *t*-distribution

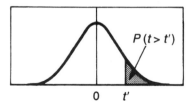

One–way probability

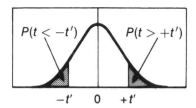

Two–way probability

To be significant, the calculated value of *t* must be greater than the critical value given in the table at the appropriate level for a given number of degrees of freedom, or less than the corresponding negative value.

	Significance level						
One-way test	0.20	0.10	0.05	0.025	0.01	0.005	0.001
Two-way test	0.40	0.20	0.10	0.05	0.02	0.01	0.002
df = 1	1.376	3.078	6.314	12.706	31.821	63.657	318.317
2	1.061	1.886	2.920	4.303	6.965	9.925	22.327
3	0.979	1.638	2.353	3.182	4.541	5.841	10.215
4	0.941	1.533	2.132	2.776	3.747	4.604	7.713
5	0.920	1.476	2.015	2.571	3.365	4.032	5.893
6	0.906	1.440	1.943	2.447	3.143	3.707	5.208
7	0.896	1.415	1.895	2.365	2.998	3.499	4.785
8	0.889	1.397	1.860	2.306	2.896	3.355	4.501
9	0.883	1.383	1.833	2.262	2.821	3.250	4.297
10	0.879	1.372	1.812	2.228	2.764	3.169	4.144
11	0.876	1.363	1.796	2.201	2.718	3.106	4.025

	Significance level						
One-way test	0.20	0.10	0.05	0.025	0.01	0.005	0.001
Two-way test	0.40	0.20	0.10	0.05	0.02	0.01	0.002
12	0.873	1.356	1.782	2.179	2.681	3.055	3.930
13	0.870	1.350	1.771	2.150	2.650	3.012	3.852
14	0.868	1.345	1.761	2.145	2.624	2.977	3.787
15	0.866	1.341	1.753	2.131	2.602	2.947	3.733
16	0.865	1.337	1.746	2.120	2.583	2.921	3.686
17	0.863	1.333	1.740	2.110	2.567	2.898	3.646
18	0.862	1.330	1.734	2.101	2.552	2.878	3.610
19	0.861	1.328	1.729	2.093	2.539	2.861	3.579
20	0.860	1.325	1.725	2.086	2.528	2.845	3.552
21	0.859	1.323	1.721	2.080	2.518	2.831	3.527
22	0.858	1.321	1.717	2.074	2.508	2.819	3.505
23	0.858	1.319	1.714	2.069	2.500	2.807	3.485
24	0.857	1.318	1.711	2.064	2.492	2.797	3.467
25	0.856	1.316	1.708	2.060	2.485	2.787	3.450
26	0.856	1.315	1.706	2.056	2.479	2.779	3.435
27	0.855	1.314	1.703	2.052	2.473	2.771	3.421
28	0.855	1.313	1.701	2.048	2.467	2.763	3.408
29	0.854	1.311	1.699	2.045	2.462	2.756	3.396
30	0.854	1.310	1.697	2.042	2.457	2.750	3.385
40	0.851	1.303	1.684	2.021	2.423	2.704	3.307
60	0.848	1.296	1.671	2.000	2.390	2.660	3.232
120	0.845	1.289	1.658	1.980	2.358	2.617	3.160
INF	0.842	1.282	1.645	1.960	2.326	2.576	3.090

Table C   Critical values of the chi-square distribution

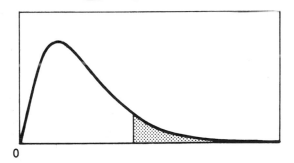

0

To be significant, the calculated value of χ^2 must be larger than the critical value given in the table at the appropriate level.

Note that a one-way test is possible in the case of a 2×2 contingency table whereupon the significance level for a given critical value of χ^2 is halved.

	\multicolumn{6}{c}{Significance level}					
	0.20	0.10	0.05	0.025	0.01	0.005
df = 1	1.64	2.71	3.84	5.02	6.64	7.88
2	3.22	4.61	5.99	7.38	9.21	10.60
3	4.64	6.25	7.82	9.35	11.34	12.84
4	5.99	7.78	9.49	11.14	13.28	14.86
5	7.29	9.24	11.07	12.83	15.09	16.75
6	8.56	10.64	12.59	14.45	16.81	18.55
7	9.80	12.02	14.07	16.01	18.48	20.28
8	11.03	13.36	15.51	17.53	20.09	21.95
9	12.24	14.68	16.92	19.02	21.67	23.59
10	13.44	15.99	18.31	20.48	23.21	25.19
11	14.63	17.28	19.68	21.92	24.72	26.76
12	15.81	18.55	21.03	23.34	26.22	28.30
13	16.98	19.81	22.36	24.74	27.69	29.82
14	18.15	21.06	23.68	26.12	29.14	31.32
15	19.31	22.31	25.00	27.49	30.58	32.80
16	20.47	23.54	26.30	28.85	32.00	34.27
17	21.61	24.77	27.59	30.19	33.41	35.72
18	22.76	25.99	28.87	31.53	34.81	37.16
19	23.90	27.20	30.14	32.85	36.19	38.58
20	25.04	28.41	31.41	34.17	37.57	40.00
21	26.17	29.62	32.67	35.48	38.93	41.40
22	27.30	30.81	33.92	36.78	40.29	42.80
23	28.43	32.01	35.17	38.08	41.64	44.18
24	29.55	33.20	36.42	39.36	42.98	45.56
25	30.68	34.38	37.65	40.65	44.31	46.93
26	31.79	35.56	38.89	41.92	45.64	48.29
27	32.91	36.74	40.11	43.19	46.96	49.64
28	34.03	37.92	41.34	44.46	48.28	50.99
29	35.14	39.09	42.56	45.72	49.59	52.34
30	36.25	40.26	43.77	46.98	50.89	53.67

Table D   Critical values of the F-distribution

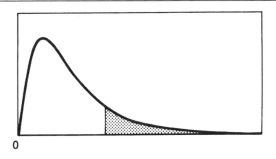

0

For the calculated value of F to be significant, it should exceed the value quoted in the table at the accepted level of significance for the appropriate numbers of degrees of freedom for each sample. The values quoted, at the 5%, 2.5% and 1% levels, correspond to a one-tailed or directional probability as would be required in an ANOVA. In the case of a two-way test, as would be the case when comparing the precision, i.e. the variance or standard deviation, of two sets of measurements, the significance level should be halved.

For convenience, values of F less than unity are not quoted so, except in the case of the ANOVA, the calculated value is obtained by placing the larger variance estimate in the numerator so that F always exceeds unity.

Number of degrees of freedom of the larger variance estimate df_1

		1	2	3	4	5	6	7	8	9	12	24	INF
$df_2 = 1$	0.05	161.4	199.5	215.7	224.6	230.2	234	236.8	238.9	240.5	243.9	249.1	254.3
	0.025	617.8	799.5	864.2	899.6	921.8	937.1	748.2	956.7	963.3	976.7	997.2	1081
	0.01	4052	4999	5403	5625	5764	5859	5928	5981	6020	6106	6235	6366
2	0.05	18.51	19.00	19.16	19.25	19.30	19.33	19.35	19.37	19.38	19.41	19.45	19.50
	0.025	38.51	39.00	39.17	39.25	39.30	39.33	39.36	39.37	39.39	39.41	39.46	39.50
	0.01	98.50	99.00	99.17	99.25	99.30	99.33	99.36	2.68	99.39	99.42	99.46	99.50
3	0.05	10.13	9.55	9.28	9.12	9.01	8.94	8.89	8.85	8.81	8.75	8.64	8.53
	0.025	17.40	16.04	15.44	15.10	14.88	14.73	14.62	14.54	14.47	14.34	14.12	13.90
	0.01	34.12	30.82	28.46	28.71	28.24	27.91	27.67	27.49	27.34	27.05	26.60	26.13
4	0.05	7.71	6.94	6.59	6.39	6.26	6.16	6.09	6.04	5.60	5.91	5.77	5.63
	0.025	12.22	10.65	9.98	9.60	9.36	9.20	9.07	8.98	8.90	8.75	8.51	8.26
	0.01	21.20	18.00	16.69	15.98	15.52	15.21	14.98	14.80	14.66	14.37	13.93	13.46

(continued)

Table D *(continued)*

Number of degrees of freedom of the larger variance estimate df_1

		1	2	3	4	5	6	7	8	9	12	24	INF
$df_2 = 5$	0.05	6.61	5.79	5.41	5.19	5.05	4.95	4.88	4.82	4.77	4.68	4.53	4.37
	0.025	10.01	6.43	7.76	7.39	7.15	6.98	6.85	6.76	6.68	6.52	6.28	6.02
	0.01	16.26	13.27	12.06	11.39	10.97	10.67	10.46	10.29	10.16	9.89	9.47	9.02
6	0.05	5.99	5.14	4.76	4.53	4.39	4.28	4.21	4.15	4.10	3.00	3.84	3.67
	0.025	8.81	7.26	6.60	6.23	5.99	5.82	5.70	5.60	5.52	5.37	5.12	4.85
	0.01	13.74	10.92	9.78	9.15	8.75	8.47	8.26	8.10	7.98	7.72	7.31	6.88
7	0.05	5.59	4.74	4.35	4.12	3.97	3.87	3.79	3.73	3.68	3.58	3.41	3.23
	0.025	8.07	6.54	5.89	5.52	5.29	5.12	4.99	4.90	4.82	4.67	4.42	4.14
	0.01	12.25	9.55	8.45	7.85	7.46	7.19	6.99	6.84	6.72	6.47	6.07	5.65
8	0.05	5.32	4.46	4.07	3.84	3.69	3.58	3.50	3.44	3.39	3.28	3.12	2.93
	0.025	7.57	6.06	5.42	5.05	4.82	4.65	4.53	4.43	4.36	4.20	3.95	3.67
	0.01	11.26	8.65	7.59	7.01	6.63	6.37	6.18	6.03	5.91	5.67	5.28	4.86
9	0.05	5.18	4.26	3.86	3.63	3.48	3.37	3.29	3.23	3.18	3.07	2.90	2.71
	0.025	7.21	5.71	5.08	4.72	4.48	4.32	4.20	4.10	4.03	3.87	3.61	3.33
	0.01	10.56	8.02	6.99	6.42	6.06	5.80	5.61	5.47	5.35	5.11	4.73	4.31
10	0.05	4.96	4.10	3.71	3.48	3.33	3.22	3.14	3.07	3.02	2.91	2.74	2.54
	0.025	6.94	5.46	4.83	4.47	4.24	4.07	3.95	3.85	3.38	3.62	3.37	3.06
	0.01	10.04	7.56	6.55	5.99	5.64	5.39	5.20	5.06	4.94	4.71	4.33	3.91
11	0.05	4.84	3.98	3.59	3.36	3.20	3.09	3.01	3.95	3.90	2.79	2.61	2.40
	0.025	6.72	5.26	4.63	4.28	4.04	3.88	3.76	3.66	3.59	3.43	3.17	2.88
	0.01	9.65	7.21	6.22	5.67	5.32	5.07	4.89	4.74	4.63	4.40	4.02	3.60
12	0.05	4.75	3.89	3.49	3.26	3.11	3.00	2.91	2.85	3.80	2.69	2.51	2.30
	0.025	6.55	5.10	4.47	4.12	3.89	3.73	3.61	3.51	3.44	3.28	3.02	2.72
	0.01	9.33	6.93	5.95	5.41	5.06	4.82	4.64	4.50	4.39	4.16	3.78	3.36
13	0.05	4.67	3.81	3.41	3.18	3.03	2.92	2.83	2.77	2.71	2.60	2.42	2.21
	0.025	6.41	4.97	4.35	4.00	3.77	3.60	3.48	3.39	3.31	3.15	2.89	2.60
	0.01	9.07	6.70	5.74	5.21	4.86	4.62	4.44	4.30	4.23	3.96	3.59	3.17
14	0.05	4.60	3.74	3.34	3.11	2.96	2.85	2.76	2.70	2.65	2.53	2.35	2.13
	0.025	6.30	4.86	4.24	3.89	3.66	3.50	3.38	3.29	3.21	3.05	2.79	2.49
	0.01	8.86	6.51	5.56	5.04	4.70	4.46	4.28	4.14	4.03	3.80	3.43	3.00
15	0.05	4.54	3.68	3.29	3.06	2.90	2.79	2.71	2.64	2.59	2.48	2.29	2.07
	0.025	6.20	4.76	4.15	3.80	3.58	3.41	3.29	3.20	3.12	2.96	2.70	2.40
	0.01	8.68	6.36	5.42	4.89	4.56	4.32	4.14	4.00	3.89	3.67	3.29	2.87
16	0.05	4.49	3.63	3.24	3.01	2.85	2.74	2.66	2.59	2.54	2.42	2.24	2.01
	0.025	6.12	4.69	4.08	3.73	3.50	3.34	3.22	3.12	3.05	2.69	2.63	2.32
	0.01	8.53	6.23	5.29	4.77	4.44	4.20	4.03	3.89	3.78	3.55	3.18	2.75

Number of degrees of freedom of the larger variance estimate df_1

		1	2	3	4	5	6	7	8	9	12	24	INF
$df_2 = 17$	0.05	4.45	3.59	3.20	2.96	2.81	2.70	2.61	2.55	2.49	2.38	2.19	1.96
	0.025	6.04	4.62	4.01	3.66	3.44	3.28	3.16	3.06	2.98	2.82	2.56	2.25
	0.01	8.40	6.11	5.18	4.67	4.34	4.10	3.93	3.79	3.68	3.46	3.08	2.65
18	0.05	4.41	3.55	3.16	2.93	2.77	2.66	2.68	2.51	2.46	2.34	2.15	1.92
	0.025	5.98	4.56	3.95	3.61	3.38	3.22	3.10	3.01	2.93	2.77	2.50	2.19
	0.01	8.29	6.01	5.09	4.58	4.25	4.01	3.84	3.71	3.60	3.37	3.00	2.57
19	0.05	4.38	3.52	3.13	2.90	2.74	2.63	2.54	2.48	2.42	2.31	2.11	1.88
	0.025	5.92	4.51	3.90	3.56	3.33	3.17	3.05	2.96	2.88	2.72	2.45	2.13
	0.01	8.18	5.93	5.01	4.50	4.17	3.94	3.77	3.63	3.52	3.30	2.92	2.49
20	0.05	4.35	3.49	3.10	2.87	2.71	2.60	2.51	2.45	2.39	2.28	2.08	1.84
	0.025	5.87	4.46	3.86	3.51	3.29	3.13	3.01	2.91	2.84	2.68	2.41	2.09
	0.01	8.10	5.85	4.94	4.43	4.10	3.87	3.70	3.56	3.46	3.23	2.86	2.42
21	0.05	4.32	3.47	3.07	2.84	2.68	2.57	2.49	2.42	2.37	2.25	2.05	1.81
	0.025	5.83	4.42	3.82	3.48	3.25	3.09	2.97	2.87	2.80	2.64	2.37	2.04
	0.01	8.02	5.78	4.87	4.37	4.04	3.81	3.64	3.51	3.40	3.17	2.80	2.36
22	0.05	4.30	3.44	3.05	2.82	2.66	2.55	2.45	2.40	2.34	2.23	2.03	1.78
	0.025	5.79	4.38	3.78	3.44	3.22	3.05	2.93	2.84	2.76	2.60	2.33	2.00
	0.01	7.95	5.72	4.82	4.31	3.99	3.76	3.59	3.45	3.35	3.12	2.75	2.31
23	0.05	4.28	3.42	3.03	2.80	2.64	2.53	2.44	2.37	2.32	2.20	2.00	1.76
	0.025	5.76	4.35	3.75	3.41	3.18	3.02	2.90	2.81	2.73	2.57	2.30	1.97
	0.01	7.88	5.66	4.76	4.26	3.94	3.71	3.54	3.41	3.30	3.07	2.70	2.26
24	0.05	4.26	3.40	3.01	2.78	2.62	2.51	2.42	2.36	2.30	2.18	1.98	1.73
	0.025	5.72	4.32	3.72	3.38	3.15	2.99	2.87	2.78	2.70	2.54	2.27	1.94
	0.01	7.82	5.61	4.72	4.22	3.90	3.67	3.50	3.36	3.26	3.03	2.66	2.21
25	0.05	4.24	3.39	2.99	2.76	2.60	2.49	2.40	2.34	2.82	2.16	1.96	1.71
	0.025	5.69	4.29	3.69	3.35	3.13	2.97	2.85	2.75	2.68	2.51	2.24	1.91
	0.01	7.77	5.57	4.68	4.18	3.86	3.63	3.46	3.32	3.22	2.99	2.62	2.17
26	0.05	4.23	3.37	2.98	2.74	2.59	2.47	2.39	2.32	2.27	2.15	1.95	1.69
	0.025	5.66	4.27	3.67	3.33	3.10	2.94	2.82	2.73	2.65	2.49	2.22	1.88
	0.01	7.72	5.53	4.64	4.14	3.82	3.59	3.42	3.29	3.18	2.96	2.58	2.13
27	0.05	4.21	3.35	2.96	2.73	2.57	2.46	2.37	2.31	2.25	2.13	1.93	1.67
	0.025	5.63	4.24	3.65	3.31	3.08	2.92	2.80	2.71	2.63	2.47	2.19	1.85
	0.01	7.68	5.49	4.60	4.11	3.78	3.56	3.39	3.26	3.15	2.93	2.55	2.10
28	0.05	4.20	3.34	2.95	2.71	2.56	2.45	2.36	2.29	2.24	2.12	1.91	1.65
	0.025	5.61	4.22	3.63	3.29	3.06	2.90	2.78	2.69	2.61	2.45	2.17	1.83
	0.01	7.64	5.45	4.57	4.07	3.75	3.53	3.36	3.23	3.12	2.90	2.52	2.06

(continued)

Table D *(continued)*

Number of degrees of freedom of the larger variance estimate df_1

		1	2	3	4	5	6	7	8	9	12	24	INF
$df_2 = 29$	0.05	4.18	3.33	2.93	2.70	2.55	2.43	2.35	2.28	2.22	2.10	1.90	1.64
	0.025	5.59	4.20	3.61	3.27	3.04	2.88	2.76	2.67	2.59	2.43	2.15	1.81
	0.01	7.60	5.42	4.54	4.04	3.73	3.50	3.33	3.20	3.09	2.87	2.49	2.03
30	0.05	4.17	3.32	2.92	2.69	2.53	2.42	2.33	2.27	2.21	2.09	1.89	1.62
	0.025	5.57	4.18	3.59	3.25	3.03	2.87	2.75	2.65	2.57	2.41	2.14	1.79
	0.01	7.56	5.39	4.51	4.02	3.70	3.47	3.30	3.17	3.07	2.84	2.47	2.01
40	0.05	4.08	3.23	2.84	2.61	2.45	2.34	2.25	2.18	2.12	2.00	1.79	1.51
	0.025	5.42	4.05	3.46	3.13	2.90	2.74	2.62	2.53	2.45	2.29	2.01	1.64
	0.01	7.31	5.18	4.31	3.83	3.51	3.29	3.12	2.99	2.89	2.66	2.29	1.80
50	0.05	4.00	3.15	2.76	2.53	2.37	2.25	2.17	2.10	2.04	1.92	1.70	1.39
	0.025	5.29	3.93	3.34	3.01	2.79	2.63	2.51	2.41	2.33	2.17	1.88	1.48
	0.01	7.08	4.98	4.13	3.65	3.34	3.12	2.95	2.82	2.72	2.50	2.12	1.60
120	0.05	3.92	3.07	2.68	2.45	2.29	2.18	2.09	2.02	1.96	1.83	1.61	1.25
	0.025	5.15	3.80	3.23	2.89	2.67	2.52	2.39	2.30	2.22	2.05	1.76	1.31
	0.01	6.85	4.79	3.95	3.48	3.17	2.96	2.79	2.66	2.56	2.34	1.95	1.38
INF	0.05	3.84	3.00	2.60	2.37	2.21	2.10	2.01	2.94	1.88	1.75	1.52	1.01
	0.025	5.02	3.69	3.12	2.79	2.57	2.41	2.29	2.19	2.12	1.94	1.64	1.00
	0.01	6.63	4.61	3.78	3.32	3.02	2.80	2.64	2.51	2.42	2.18	1.79	1.00

Table E   Critical values of the Mann–Whitney distribution

To be significant in either a two-way or a one-way test, the smaller of the two calculated values of U must be equal to, or less than, the tabulated value at the appropriate significance level for the sample sizes n_1 and n_2.

ONE-WAY TEST $P = 0.05$
TWO-WAY TEST $P = 0.10$

$n_1 =$	2	3	4	5	6	7	8	9	10	11	12	13	14	15	16	17	18	19	20
$n_2 = 2$	–	–	–	0	0	0	1	1	1	1	2	2	2	3	3	3	4	4	4
3	–	0	0	1	2	2	3	3	4	5	5	6	7	7	8	9	9	10	11
4	–	0	1	2	3	4	5	6	7	8	9	10	11	12	14	15	16	17	18
5	0	1	2	4	5	6	8	9	11	12	13	15	16	18	19	20	22	23	25
6	0	2	3	5	7	8	10	12	14	16	17	19	21	23	25	26	28	30	32
7	0	2	4	6	8	11	13	15	17	19	21	24	26	28	30	33	35	37	39

$n_1 =$	2	3	4	5	6	7	8	9	10	11	12	13	14	15	16	17	18	19	20
$n_2 = 8$	1	3	5	8	10	13	15	18	20	23	26	28	31	33	36	39	41	44	47
9	1	3	6	9	12	15	18	21	24	27	30	33	36	39	42	45	48	51	54
10	1	4	7	11	14	17	20	24	27	31	34	37	41	44	48	51	55	58	62
11	1	5	8	12	16	19	23	27	31	34	38	42	46	50	54	57	61	65	69
12	2	5	9	13	17	21	26	30	34	38	42	47	51	55	60	64	68	72	77
13	2	6	10	15	19	24	28	33	37	42	47	51	56	61	65	70	75	80	84
14	2	7	11	16	21	26	31	36	41	46	51	56	61	66	71	77	82	87	92
15	3	7	12	18	23	28	33	39	44	50	55	61	66	72	77	83	89	95	101
16	3	8	14	19	25	30	36	42	48	54	60	65	71	77	83	89	96	102	109
17	3	9	15	20	26	33	39	45	51	57	64	70	77	83	89	96	102	109	116
18	4	9	16	22	28	35	41	48	55	61	68	75	82	88	95	102	109	116	123
19	4	10	17	23	30	37	44	51	58	65	72	80	87	94	101	109	116	123	130
20	4	11	18	25	32	39	47	54	62	69	77	84	92	100	107	115	123	130	138

ONE-WAY TEST $P = 0.025$
TWO-WAY TEST $P = 0.05$

$n_1 =$	2	3	4	5	6	7	8	9	10	11	12	13	14	15	16	17	18	19	20
$n_2 = 2$	–	–	–	–	–	–	0	0	0	0	1	1	1	1	1	2	2	2	2
3	–	–	–	0	1	1	2	2	3	3	4	4	5	5	6	6	7	7	8
4	–	–	0	1	2	3	4	4	5	6	7	8	9	10	11	11	12	13	13
5	–	0	1	2	3	5	6	7	8	9	11	12	13	14	15	17	18	19	20
6	–	1	2	3	5	6	8	10	11	13	14	16	17	19	21	22	24	25	27
7	–	1	3	5	6	8	10	12	14	16	18	20	22	24	26	28	30	32	34
8	0	2	4	6	8	10	13	15	17	19	22	24	26	29	31	34	36	38	41
9	0	2	4	7	10	12	15	17	20	23	26	28	31	34	37	39	42	45	48
10	0	3	5	8	11	14	17	20	23	26	29	33	36	39	42	45	48	52	55
11	0	3	6	9	13	16	19	23	26	30	33	37	40	44	47	51	55	58	62
12	1	4	7	11	14	18	22	26	29	33	37	41	45	49	53	57	61	65	69
13	1	4	8	12	16	20	24	28	33	37	41	45	50	54	59	63	67	72	76
14	1	5	9	13	17	22	26	31	36	40	45	50	55	59	64	67	74	78	83
15	1	5	10	14	19	24	29	34	39	44	49	54	59	64	70	75	80	85	90
16	1	6	11	15	21	26	31	37	42	47	53	59	64	70	75	81	86	92	98
17	2	6	11	17	22	28	34	39	45	51	57	63	67	75	81	87	93	99	105
18	2	7	12	18	24	30	36	42	48	55	61	67	74	80	86	93	99	106	112
19	2	7	13	19	25	32	38	45	52	58	65	72	78	85	92	99	106	113	119
20	2	8	13	20	27	34	41	48	55	62	69	76	83	90	98	105	112	119	127

ONE-WAY TEST $P = 0.01$
TWO-WAY TEST $P = 0.02$

$n_1 =$	2	3	4	5	6	7	8	9	10	11	12	13	14	15	16	17	18	19	20
$n_2 = 2$	–	–	–	–	–	–	–	–	–	–	–	–	0	0	0	0	0	1	1
3	–	–	–	–	–	–	0	0	1	1	1	2	2	2	3	3	4	4	5

(continued)

Table E *(continued)*

ONE-WAY TEST $P = 0.01$ *(continued)*
TWO-WAY TEST $P = 0.02$

$n_1 =$	2	3	4	5	6	7	8	9	10	11	12	13	14	15	16	17	18	19	20
$n_2 = 4$	–	–	–	0	1	1	2	3	3	4	5	5	6	7	7	8	9	9	10
5	–	–	0	1	2	3	4	5	6	7	8	9	10	11	12	13	14	15	16
6	–	–	1	2	3	4	6	7	8	9	11	12	13	15	16	18	19	20	22
7	–	0	1	3	4	6	7	9	11	12	14	16	17	19	21	23	24	26	28
8	–	0	2	4	6	7	9	11	13	15	17	20	22	24	26	28	30	32	34
9	–	1	3	5	7	9	11	14	16	18	21	23	26	28	31	33	36	38	40
10	–	1	3	6	8	11	13	16	19	22	24	27	30	33	36	38	41	44	47
11	–	1	4	7	9	12	15	18	22	25	28	31	34	37	41	44	47	50	53
12	–	2	5	8	11	14	17	21	24	28	31	35	38	42	46	49	53	56	60
13	0	2	5	9	12	16	20	23	27	31	35	39	43	47	51	55	59	63	67
14	0	2	6	10	13	17	22	26	30	34	38	43	47	51	56	60	65	69	73
15	0	3	7	11	15	19	24	28	33	37	42	47	51	56	61	66	70	75	80
16	0	3	7	12	16	21	26	31	36	41	46	51	56	61	66	71	76	82	87
17	0	4	8	13	18	23	28	33	38	44	49	55	60	66	71	77	82	88	93
18	0	4	9	14	19	24	30	36	41	47	53	59	65	70	76	82	88	94	100
19	1	4	9	15	20	26	32	38	44	50	56	63	69	75	82	88	94	101	107
20	1	5	10	16	22	28	34	40	47	53	50	67	73	80	87	93	100	107	114

Table F   Critical values of the Wilcoxon signed-rank distribution

To be significant, the smaller value of the sum of the ranks, W, must be equal to or less than the tabulated critical value at the appropriate significance level, where n is the number of pairs of observations, ignoring any which are equal.

	Significance level				
One-way test	0.05	0.025	0.01	0.005	0.001
Two-way test	0.10	0.05	0.02	0.01	0.002
$n = 5$	0	–	–	–	–
6	2	0	–	–	–
7	3	2	0	–	–
8	5	3	1	0	–
9	8	5	3	1	–

	Significance level				
One-way test	0.05	0.025	0.01	0.005	0.001
Two-way test	0.10	0.05	0.02	0.01	0.002
$n = 10$	10	8	5	3	0
11	13	10	7	5	1
12	17	13	9	7	2
13	21	17	12	9	4
14	25	21	15	12	6
15	30	25	19	15	8
16	35	29	23	19	11
17	41	34	27	23	14
18	47	40	32	27	18
19	53	46	37	32	21
20	60	52	43	37	26
21	67	58	49	42	30
22	75	65	55	48	35
23	83	73	62	54	40
24	91	81	69	61	45
25	100	89	76	68	51
26	110	98	84	75	58
27	119	107	92	83	64
28	130	116	101	91	71
29	140	126	110	100	79
30	151	137	120	109	86
31	163	147	130	118	94
32	175	159	140	128	103
33	187	170	151	138	112
34	200	182	162	148	121
35	213	195	173	159	131
36	227	208	185	171	141
37	241	221	198	182	151
38	256	235	211	194	162
39	271	249	224	207	173
40	286	264	238	220	185

Table G   Critical values of the Pearson (product moment) correlation coefficient r

The null hypothesis is that there is no correlation ($H_0 : \rho = 0$). The correlation is significant if r exceeds the tabulated value for the appropriate number of pairs of observations (n). A one-way test is conducted if the experimental hypothesis asserts that the coefficient has a particular sign (either $H_1: \rho >$ zero or $H_1: \rho <$ zero). Note that the number of degrees of freedom, if required, is given by $(n - 2)$.

	Significance level				
One-way test	0.05	0.025	0.01	0.005	0.001
Two-way test	0.10	0.05	0.02	0.01	0.002
$n = 4$	0.900	0.950	0.980	0.990	0.998
5	0.805	0.878	0.934	0.959	0.986
6	0.729	0.811	0.882	0.917	0.963
7	0.669	0.755	0.833	0.875	0.935
8	0.622	0.707	0.789	0.834	0.905
9	0.582	0.666	0.750	0.798	0.875
10	0.549	0.632	0.716	0.765	0.847
11	0.521	0.602	0.685	0.735	0.820
12	0.497	0.576	0.658	0.708	0.795
13	0.476	0.553	0.634	0.684	0.772
14	0.458	0.532	0.612	0.661	0.750
15	0.441	0.514	0.592	0.641	0.730
16	0.426	0.497	0.574	0.623	0.711
17	0.412	0.482	0.558	0.606	0.694
18	0.400	0.468	0.543	0.590	0.678
19	0.389	0.456	0.529	0.575	0.662
20	0.378	0.444	0.516	0.561	0.648
21	0.369	0.433	0.503	0.549	0.635
22	0.360	0.423	0.492	0.537	0.622
23	0.352	0.413	0.482	0.526	0.610
24	0.344	0.404	0.472	0.515	0.599
25	0.337	0.396	0.462	0.505	0.588
26	0.330	0.388	0.453	0.496	0.578
27	0.323	0.381	0.445	0.487	0..568
28	0.317	0.374	0.437	0.479	0.559
29	0.312	0.367	0.430	0.471	0.550
30	0.306	0.361	0.423	0.463	0.542
35	0.283	0.334	0.392	0.430	0.505
40	0.264	0.312	0.367	0.403	0.474
45	0.248	0.294	0.346	0.380	0.449
50	0.235	0.279	0.328	0.361	0.427
55	0.224	0.266	0.313	0.345	0.408
60	0.214	0.254	0.300	0.330	0.391

Table H   Critical values of the Spearman rank correlation coefficient

To be significant, the value the Spearman coefficient (r_s) must be larger than the tabulated value, or smaller than the negative of the tabulated value.

$n =$ the number of pairs of observation being ranked,

	Significance level			
One-way test	0.05	0.025	0.01	0.005
Two-way test	0.10	0.05	0.02	0.01
$n = 5$	0.900	–	–	–
6	0.829	0.886	0.943	–
7	0.714	0.786	0.893	–
8	0.643	0.738	0.833	0.881
9	0.600	0.683	0.783	0.833
10	0.564	0.648	0.745	0.794
11	0.523	0.623	0.736	0.781
12	0.497	0.591	0.703	0.777
13	0.475	0.566	0.673	0.745
14	0.457	0.545	0.646	0.716
15	0.441	0.525	0.623	0.689
16	0.425	0.507	0.601	0.666
17	0.412	0.490	0.582	0.645
18	0.399	0.476	0.564	0.625
19	0.388	0.462	0.549	0.608
20	0.377	0.450	0.534	0.591
21	0.368	0.438	0.521	0.576
22	0.359	0.428	0.508	0.562
23	0.351	0.418	0.496	0.549
24	0.343	0.409	0.486	0.537
25	0.336	0.400	0.475	0.526
26	0.329	0.392	0.465	0.515
27	0.323	0.385	0.456	0.505
28	0.317	0.377	0.448	0.496
29	0.311	0.370	0.440	0.487
30	0.305	0.364	0.432	0.478

Table I   Critical values of Kendall's coefficient of concordance

For the agreement between the rankings assigned by the assessors to be significant, W should exceed the tabulated value for the relevant values of n and k at the appropriate significance level.

$k =$ the number of assessors or groups of data,

$n =$ the number of subjects being ranked.

		$n = 3$	4	5	6	7
Critical values of W	$k = 3$	–	–	0.716	0.660	0.624
	4	–	0.619	0.553	0.512	0.484
	5	–	0.501	0.449	0.417	0.395
	6	–	0.421	0.378	0.351	0.333
$P = 0.05$	8	0.376	0.318	0.287	0.267	0.253
	10	0.300	0.256	0.231	0.215	0.204
	15	0.200	0.171	0.155	0.145	0.137
	20	0.150	0.129	0.117	0.109	0.103

		$n = 3$	4	5	6	7
Critical values of W	$k = 3$	–	–	0.840	0.780	0.737
	4	–	0.768	0.683	0.629	0.592
	5	–	0.644	0.571	0.524	0.491
	6	–	0.553	0.489	0.448	0.419
$P = 0.01$	8	0.522	0.429	0.379	0.347	0.324
	10	0.426	0.351	0.309	0.282	0.263
	15	0.291	0.240	0.211	0.193	0.179
	20	0.221	0.182	0.160	0.146	0.136

Table J   Critical values of M for the Friedman test

To be significant at the level indicated by P, the calculated value of M must be larger than the critical value given in the table for the appropriate values of k and n.

If n is large the distribution of M is approximated by χ^2 and critical values may be obtained from the χ^2 distribution (Table C) at $(k - 1)$ degrees of freedom. These are shown in this table at $n =$ INF (infinity).

k = the number of different conditions under which the repeated measures, which are ranked for each subject, are taken,

n = the number of subjects of which repeated measures are taken.

$k = 3$	Significance level			
	0.10	0.05	0.025	0.01
$n = 3$	6.00	6.00	–	–
4	6.00	6.50	8.00	8.00
5	5.20	6.40	7.60	8.40
6	5.33	7.00	8.33	9.00
7	5.43	7.14	7.71	8.86
8	5.25	6.25	7.75	9.00
9	5.56	6.22	8.00	9.56
10	5.00	6.20	7.80	9.60
11	5.09	6.55	7.82	9.46
12	5.17	6.50	8.00	9.50
13	4.77	6.62	7.54	9.39
14	5.14	6.14	7.43	9.14
15	4.03	6.40	7.60	8.93
INF	4.61	5.99	7.38	9.21

$k = 4$	Significance level			
	0.10	0.05	0.025	0.01
$n = 2$	6.00	6.00	–	–
3	6.60	7.40	8.20	9.00
4	6.30	7.80	8.40	9.60
5	6.36	7.80	8.76	9.96
6	6.40	7.60	8.80	10.20
7	6.43	7.80	9.00	10.54
8	6.30	7.65	9.00	10.50
INF	6.25	7.82	9.35	11.34

$k = 5$	Significance level			
	0.10	0.05	0.025	0.01
$n = 2$	7.20	7.60	8.00	8.00
3	7.47	8.53	9.60	10.13
4	7.60	8.80	9.80	11.20
5	7.68	8.96	10.24	11.68
6	7.73	9.07	10.40	11.87
7	7.77	9.14	10.51	12.11
8	7.70	9.20	10.60	12.30
INF	7.78	9.49	11.14	13.28

$k = 6$	Significance level			
	0.10	0.05	0.025	0.01
$n = 2$	8.29	9.14	9.43	9.71
3	8.71	9.86	10.81	11.76
4	9.00	10.29	11.43	12.71
5	9.00	10.49	11.74	13.23
6	9.05	10.57	12.00	13.62
INF	9.24	11.07	12.83	15.09

Answers Section

Answers for Chapter 1

Answer 1.1

(a) These data represent a sample because the marks of only eight students from a class of 85 are given, therefore σ_{n-1} or s on the calculator should be used to calculate the standard deviation. The results quoted to one decimal place are as follows:

$$\bar{x} = 59.4 \quad s = 11.8 \quad CV = 19.8\%$$

(b) In this case we are dealing with a population because there are only ten students in the class. Therefore the σ_n or σ button on the calculator should be used.

$$\mu = 63.0 \quad \sigma = 11.2 \quad CV = 17.8\%$$

Answer 1.2

Use the σ_{n-1} button on your calculator

$$\bar{x}_1 = \bar{x}_2 = 34.7 \quad s_1 = 8.84$$

$$CV_1 = \frac{8.84}{34.7} \times 100 = 25.5\%$$

$$s_2 = 1.72$$

$$CV_1 = \frac{1.72}{34.7} \times 100 = 5.0\%$$

The second sample is more precise because it has a smaller standard deviation and, of course, coefficient of variation. Remember that precision is a measure of reproducibility and a small standard deviation indicates low variability, i.e. a high reproducibility or precision.

Answer 1.3

(a) The mean, median and (sample) standard deviation are 25.75, 25.5 and 3.24, respectively. Note that the mean and median are very close to each other. This indicates that the distribution, or spread of the data, is fairly symmetrical about the centre.

(b) The mean and standard deviation now become 30.75 and 14.61, respectively. The median remains at 25.5, which is a rather more characteristic value for these data as a whole than the new mean, which is strongly influenced by the extreme value, 66. The mean and standard deviation for the first seven numbers are 25.71 and 3.50, i.e. very close to the original values.

Answer 1.4

(a) (i) $\dfrac{12}{37} \times 100 = 32.4\%$ (ii) $\dfrac{18}{37} \times 100 = 48.6\%$

(b) $\dfrac{(18 - 12)}{37} \times 100 = 16.2\%$

Answer 1.5

$$\text{Median} = 8.5 \qquad s = 3.0 \qquad \sigma = 2.9$$
$$\bar{x} = 8.3 \qquad s^2 = 9.0 \qquad \sigma^2 = 8.6$$

Notes:

A quick scan of the data shows that the minimum and maximum values are 3 and 14 respectively. Thus, if the numbers within this range are listed on the left-hand side of a sheet of paper, a mark corresponding to each value can readily be added so that the frequency of occurrence of each can be established.

The following frequencies will be found:

3(1) 4(0) 5(4) 6(1) 7(2) 8(2) 9(5) 10(1) 11(1) 12(1) 13(0) 14(2)

Since we have 20 values, there is not one which occurs in the middle so we take the average of the 10th and 11th, i.e. the average of 8 and 9, namely 8.5.

The mean and standard deviations are determined in a straightforward manner with your calculator. You will have noted, no doubt, that $(2.9)^2 = 8.41$ and not 8.6, this is because to obtain the variance, the standard deviation should be squared directly *before* rounding off to a suitable number of decimal places, i.e. $(2.930\ 443\ 652)^2 = 8.5675 \approx 8.6$.

Answer 1.6

$$\bar{x} = 25.4 \qquad s = 6.0$$

The calculation of the mean is quite straightforward:

$$\frac{\text{Total weight}}{\text{Number of objects}} = \frac{(4 \times 25) + (3 \times 15) + (7 \times 30)}{(4 + 3 + 7)} = 25.4$$

Alternatively, most calculators may be used to obtain the mean, together with the standard deviation, by entering the following while in the SD mode:

$$25 \times 4 \text{ press } M+ \text{ button}$$

and this will enter 25 four times. Similarly

$$15 \times 3 \quad M+$$
$$30 \times 7 \quad M+$$

The mean and standard deviation may now be obtained in the usual way.

If you are unable to calculate the standard deviation in this way with your calculator the following relationship may be used (see Equation 2.5 in Chapter 2):

$$s = \sqrt{\frac{1}{n-1}\left(\sum x^2 - n\bar{x}^2\right)}$$

where:

$$\sum x^2 = (4 \times 25^2) + (3 \times 17^2) + (7 \times 30^2) = 9,475$$

$$n\bar{x}^2 = 14 \times (25.36)^2 = 9,003.81$$

i.e.

$$s = \sqrt{\frac{1}{14-1}(9,475 - 9,003.8)} = 6.0$$

Answers for Chapter 2

Answer 2.1

(a) $\bar{x} = 19.2 \quad s = 7.1 \quad s^2 = 50.9$

Remember that when calculating the variance any 'rounding off' should be left to the final result, i e the value for the standard deviation obtained with the calculator should be squared directly:

$$(7.134\,792)^2 = 50.905\,257$$

$$\approx 50.9$$

whereas:

$$(7.1)^2 = 50.41$$
$$\approx 50.4$$

Although it would be absurd to quote the standard deviation as 7.134 792 the use of this figure to obtain the variance is clearly sensible. The value for the variance, and of course, the standard deviation, may then be rounded to the required number of decimal places.

(b)

Table 2.4   *Distribution of recovery time in a sample of patients*

Class mark	Class boundaries	Frequency	Cumulative frequency	Cumulative frequency %
10	8–12	2	2	10
14	12–16	6	8	40
18	16–20	4	12	60
22	20–24	3	15	75
26	24–28	2	17	85
30	28–32	1	18	90
34	32–36	1	19	95
38	36–40	1	20	100

Remember the convention that if an observation falls on a class boundary it is placed in the higher class.

(c) The histogram is not symmetrical, it is distinctly skewed to the right, i.e. is 'top heavy' on the left. It would therefore be concluded that this sample is unlikely to follow a normal distribution. Since the sample is so small, however, it is not possible to be sure about this.

(d) See Figure 2.6. The median is estimated at 18 days.

(e) It can also be seen from Figure 2.6 that about 63% of patients would be expected to recover within three weeks (21 days).

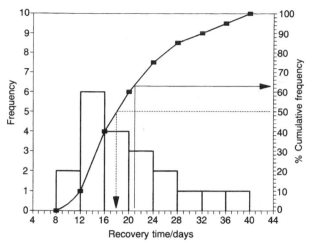

Figure 2.6 *From the histogram we can see that the median is 18 days and that 63% of patients recover from the injury within three weeks (21 days)*

Answer 2.2

(a) There are ten measurements, therefore nine degrees of freedom.

(b) The ten blood pressure measurements represent a sample, the mean of which is an estimate of the population mean. Similarly, the variance and standard deviation of the sample are estimates of the population values.

$$\bar{x} = 127.6 \text{ mmHg} \quad s^2 = 57.8 \text{ mmHg}^2 \quad s = 7.6 \text{ mmHg}$$

We shall see in Chapter 6 that a confidence level can be put on this estimate, in other words we can assess its reliability.

Answer 2.3

(a) The frequencies in each class are as follows:

Class mark	Class boundaries	Frequency	Cumulative frequency	Cumulative frequency %
108	106–110	1	1	4
112	110–114	2	3	12
116	114–118	3	6	24
120	118–122	8	14	56
124	122–126	7	21	84
128	126–130	3	24	96
132	130–134	1	25	100

(b) The cumulative frequency plot will show, when rounded to the nearest whole number:

$$\text{median} = 121$$
$$Q1 = 118$$
$$Q3 = 124$$

Thus the interquartile range (the range including the middle 50% of the observations) is 118–124.

(c) Also, from the plot, an estimate of the range, rounded to the nearest whole number, which we would expect to include 95% of the population may be obtained by drawing horizontal lines at 2.5% and 97.5% cumulative frequency, to intersect the curve at 110 and 131 respectively.

This 'reference range' (110 to 131) would be rather unreliable because the sample is so small, i.e. only 25 measurements.

Answer 2.4

From the histogram and the percentage cumulative frequency plot, the median is found to be 72 bpm and the value above which 10% of the population would be found may be estimated at a little over 82 bpm.

Remember that the cumulative frequency curve represents the value of the variable (in this case the heart rate) below which the indicated percentage of observations or measurements will be found. No measurements are found below the lower class boundary of the first class, namely 54, therefore the point corresponding to 0% is placed at that position. From the curve the value below which 90%, or above which 10%, of the observations are found can thus be determined.

Refer to p. 27 if necessary to remind yourself how to estimate the mean and standard deviation of the grouped data. These will be found to be 72.6 and 7.62 bpm respectively.

Answer 2.5

(a) $$\bar{x} = 10.2 \quad s = 1.84$$
(b) The exact nature of the histogram will depend on the choice of class boundaries, e.g.

Class boundaries	Frequency
6–7	1
7–8	2
8–9	1
9–10	4
10–11	5
11–12	4
12–13	2
13–14	1

(c) (i) 10.2

Answers for Chapter 3

Answer 3.1

Since the children were ranked by the therapists, each data set must include the integers 1 to 5 and cannot contain shared ranks. Therefore either the Pearson formula (Equation 3.2) may be applied to the ranks, or the Spearman formula (Equation 3.3) may be used.

In either case a value $r_s = 0.700$ is obtained. Once again, we would be looking for a positive correlation so we use a one-way test. Reference to Table H in Appendix VI shows that, for $n = 5$, the critical value at 5% is 0.900. Remember that the larger the value of r_s, the less likely it is that it has occurred by chance and the stronger is the correlation. Since the calculated value is less than 0.900, the probability that it has occurred by chance is greater than 5%. There is thus insufficient evidence to reject the null hypothesis (H_0: $\rho = 0$) so, by default, we are obliged to accept it and conclude that there is not a significant correlation between the two sets of data.

Answer 3.2

(a) From the appearance of the scatterplot, we can see that the relationship appears to be linear only within a limited range up to about day 25 or 29.

(b) (i) Using all the data: $r = 0.958$. It can be seen from the tables that this is a very highly significant result ($P < 0.002$). We can see, therefore, that a very highly significant correlation does not necessarily imply a linear relationship. (ii) if only the data up to day 29 are used in the calculation: $r = 0.992$. This shows an even stronger relationship.

(c) Using only the data up to day 29:

$$\text{Grip strength} = 24.0 + 0.752(\text{Days})$$

To draw the line of best fit the coordinates of two points are calculated by substituting arbitrary values for 'days' into the regression equation. It is clearly best to use one low and one high value, e.g. if day 1 is taken:

$$\text{Grip strength} = 24.0 + 0.752(1)$$
$$= 24.8$$

Similarly, considering day 29:

$$\text{Grip strength} = 24.0 + 0.752(29)$$
$$= 45.8$$

The plot, with the regression line included, may be seen in Figure 3.14.

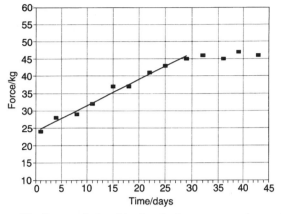

Figure 3.14 *The linear relationship clearly does not extend past about day 27*

Answer 3.3

(a) If the first measurement is assigned year $= 1$ the regression equation is as follows:

$$\text{Time} = 50.61 - 0.1659(\text{Year})$$

This equation applies only if the first value is registered at year $= 1$, when the value lying on the line of best fit is thus:

$$50.61 - 0.1659(1) = 50.44$$

The way in which the year is represented is quite arbitrary and will not alter the slope of the line, although the value of the constant will be different. For example, if the year corresponding to the first value is specified, say 1985, the equation becomes:

$$\text{Time} = 379.75 - 0.1659(\text{Specified year})$$

(b) The correlation coefficient $r = -0.892$ with eight degrees of freedom. $P < 0.001$ for a one-way correlation, i.e. very highly significant.

(c) Using the first equation obtained above and substituting Year $= 11$ we find:

$$\text{Time} = 50.61 - 0.1659(11)$$

$$= 48.76 \text{ s}$$

To obtain the value for 20 years after the last recorded time, we must substitute Year = 30:

$$\text{Time} = 50.61 - 0.1659(30)$$

$$= 45.62 \text{ s}$$

The first prediction is reasonable although, because there is rather a lot of scatter, we would not be too surprised if it is not very close to this value which represents the most probable time for the following year bearing in mind the way in which the time has reduced during the previous ten years.

The prediction for 20 years later, however, is very uncertain because we have no evidence to suggest the linear relationship observed in the first ten years will be sustained for another 20 years. If we substitute Year = 305 we find that the time is zero, which is clearly absurd.

Answer 3.4

We wish to compare ten sets of rankings of three subjects so we require Kendall's coefficient of concordance with $k = 10$ and $n = 3$.

	Ranks ($n = 3$)		
	3	1	2
	1	3	2
	3	2	1
	1	2	3
Assessors $k = 10$	1	3	2
	2	1	3
	1	2	3
	1	3	2
	3	2	1
	1	2	3
Sum of the ranks =	17	21	22

$$\text{Mean rank total} = \frac{17 + 21 + 22}{3} = 20$$

$$s = \sum (R_T - R_M)^2$$
$$= (17 - 20)^2 + (21 - 20)^2 + (22 - 20)^2$$
$$= 14$$

$$\tfrac{1}{12}k^2(n^3 - n) = \tfrac{1}{12}(10)^2(3^3 - 3) = 200$$

W may now be calculated:

$$W = \frac{14}{200}$$
$$= 0.07$$

Referring to Table I, we find the critical value at the 1% level of significance $(P = 0.01)$ for W with $k = 10$ and $n = 3$ to be 0.426. The calculated value of 0.07 is well below this so we cannot reject the null hypothesis that there is no general agreement and we must conclude that the rankings are at random, i.e. there is no particular preference for any one book by the students.

Answer 3.5

When the seven children are placed in rank order according to the number of sections answered correctly, the following was obtained:

Ranks of children ($n = 7$)

	2	5	3.5	3.5	1	6.5	6.5
Test	2	2	2	4	5.5	5.5	7
($k = 4$)	3	1	2	4.5	4.5	6	7
	1	2.5	2.5	7	4.5	4.5	6
Sum of the ranks =	8	10.5	10	19	15.5	22.5	26.5

$$\text{Mean rank total} = \frac{8 + 10.5 + 10 + 19 + 15.5 + 22.5 + 26.5}{7}$$

$$= 16$$

$$S = \sum (R_T - R_M)^2$$

$$= (8 - 16)^2 + (10.5 - 16)^2 + \cdots$$

$$+ (22.5 - 16)^2 + (26.5 - 16)^2$$

$$= 292$$

Since there are some tied ranks, the correction should be applied:

$$T_1 = \frac{(2^3 - 2) + (2^3 - 2)}{12} = 1$$

$$T_2 = \frac{(3^3 - 3) + (2^3 - 2)}{12} = 2.5$$

$$T_3 = \frac{(2^3 - 2)}{12} = 0.5$$

$$T_4 = \frac{(2^3 - 2) + (2^3 - 2)}{12} = 1$$

$$\therefore \quad \sum T = 5$$

and

$$\tfrac{1}{12} k^2 (n^3 - n) = \tfrac{1}{12}(4)^2(7^3 - 7) = 448$$

The value of W corrected for tied ranks can now be calculated:

$$W = \frac{292}{448 - k \sum T}$$

$$= 0.682$$

Referring to Table 1 we conclude that $P < 0.01$ and therefore there is significant agreement between the different tests.

Answers for Chapter 4

Answer 4.1

$$\text{The probability of requiring repair} = \frac{785}{15,600} = 0.050$$

$\therefore$ the probability of not requiring repair $= 1 - 0.050$

$$= 0.95$$

Answer 4.2

(a) In this case two values for Z are calculated:

$$Z_1 = -0.88 \quad Z_2 = +1.63$$

From Table A we see that CDF $(Z = 0.88)$ or $\phi(0.88)$ is 0.8106, thus the probability that Z will be *less* than the *positive* value $+0.88$ is 0.8106, or the probability that it will *exceed* this value is $(1 - 0.8106) = 0.1894$. Since the distribution is symmetrical, this is equal to the probability that Z will be less than -0.88, i.e. $P(Z > +0.88) = P(Z < -0.88) = 0.1894$.

We see also that $P(Z < 1.63) = 0.9484$. Thus the probability that a value of Z between these two values, -0.88 and 1.63, which is, of course, the probability that the resting pulse rate will lie between 65 and 85, is given by $(0.9484 - 0.1894) - 0.759$. It should be stressed that one *probability* is subtracted from the other and *not* the value of Z.

It is helpful, with problems of this kind, to sketch the distributions, which are shown, with the probabilities shaded, in Figure 4.11a to d.

(b) Since the probability that any person chosen at random will have a pulse rate within this range is 0.759, in a group of 625 individuals the expected number is 474, i.e. 0.759×625.

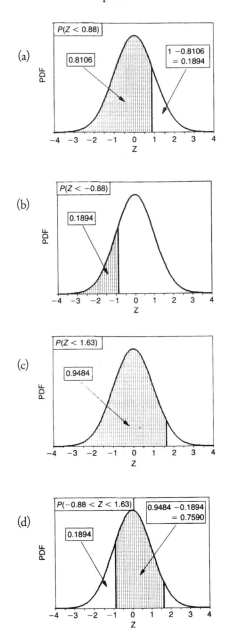

Figure 4.11a, b, c and d *The determination of the probability that* $-0.88 < Z < 1.63$.

Answer 4.3

(a) (i) $P(x > 70) = 1 - P(x < 70) = 1 - P(Z < 0.714) = 0.24$

(ii) $P(x > 80) = P(Z > 2.143) = 0.016$

(iii) $P(x > 45) = P(Z > -2.857) = 0.998$

(iv) $P(x > 65) = P(Z > 0) = 0.5$

(b) (i) 0.016   (ii) 0.67   (iii) 0.24

(c) (i) $Z_1 = -0.714$ $Z_2 = +0.714$

$P(Z < -0.714) = 0.24$ $P(Z < +0.714) = 0.76$

$\therefore$ $P(-0.714 < Z < +0.714) = 0.76 - 0.24 = 0.52$

(ii) $Z_1 = -2.143$ $Z_2 = +1.429$

$P(Z < -2.143) = 0.016$ $P(Z < +1.429) = 0.924$

$\therefore$ $P(-2.143 < Z < +1.429) = 0.924 - 0.016 = 0.91$

Remember that it is often very useful to draw a rough sketch of the distribution curve marking in the values of Z (or x) so that the relevant areas can be easily seen, e.g. for (c)(ii) the sketch shown in Figure 4.12 may be helpful.

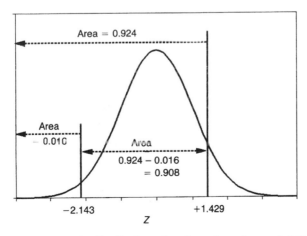

Figure 4.12 *A normal distribution showing that the probability that* $-2.143 < Z < +1.429$ *is* 0.908

Answer 4.4

(a)
$$\text{Reference range} = \mu \pm 1.96(\sigma)$$
$$= 69 \pm 1.96(4.5)$$
$$= 60.2 \text{ to } 77.8$$

(b)
$$Z = \frac{x - \mu}{\sigma} = -2.0$$

$$P(Z < -2.0) = 1 - P(Z < +2.0) = 0.023$$

i.e. 2.3% of the population would be expected to have a blood protein concentration of less than 60 g/l.

(c) The interquartile range is given by:

$$x = \mu \pm Z_{0.75}(4.5)$$

Note: $Z_{0.75}$ is the value of Z below which there is a probability of 0.75 that a random observation will fall, i.e. 75% of the population would be expected to fall below this value or 25% above this value. Similarly 25% would be expected to fall below $Z_{0.25}$, which is the same as $-Z_{0.75}$. $Z_{0.75} = 0.675$, thus the interquartile range is given by:

$$69 \pm 0.675(4.5) = 66.0 \text{ to } 72.0 \text{ g/l}$$

Answer 4.5

(a) 27.8 to 44.2
(b) 33.2 to 38.8

Answers for Chapter 5

Answer 5.1

(a) The standard error of the mean is given by:

$$\text{SE(mean)} = \sigma_{\bar{x}} = \frac{\sigma}{\sqrt{n}} = \frac{20}{\sqrt{40}} = 3.2 \text{ mmHg}$$

(b) $$Z = \frac{\bar{x} - \mu}{\sigma/\sqrt{n}} = \frac{115.8 - 120}{20/\sqrt{40}} = -1.33$$

Since we are concerned with a *reduction* in blood pressure, a one-way test is appropriate. From the tables:

$$P(Z < -1.33) = P(Z > +1.33) = 1 - P(Z < +1.33)$$
$$= 1 - 0.908 = 0.092$$

i.e. $$P = 0.092$$

Since $P > 0.05$ there is insufficient evidence to reject the null hypothesis so we must conclude that there is not a significant difference between the mean of the sample and the accepted population mean.

(c) From the tables we can see that $Z = -1.645$ to exclude 5% in the left-hand tail of the distribution. From the definition of Z we can write:

$$\bar{x} = \mu + Z(\sigma/\sqrt{n}) = 120 + (-1.645)(20/\sqrt{40}) = 114.8 \text{ mmHg}$$

Answer 5.2

We are looking for a *difference* between the means, thus a two-way test is appropriate.

$$SE(\text{mean}) = 9.8/\sqrt{39} = 1.57$$

$$Z = 2.10; \quad P(Z > 2.10) = 1 - P(Z < 2.10)$$
$$= 1 - 0.982 = 0.018$$

i.e. the sample mean differs from the population mean by 2.1 standard errors. The probability that it will take a value of 2.1 standard errors above the mean by chance is 0.018, and the probability that it will take a value of 2.1 standard errors below the mean is also 0.018. Thus, the probability that it will *differ* from the mean by 2.1 standard errors is $2 \times 0.018 = 0.036$, i.e.

$$P = 0.036$$

There is only a 3.6% probability that the observed difference would occur by chance if the true mean of the sample is the same as the population mean (the null hypothesis is true), and since this is less than 5%, we therefore conclude that the difference is significant.

Answer 5.3

(a)

$$\text{SE(mean)} = \sigma_{\bar{x}} = \frac{\sigma}{\sqrt{n}} = \frac{5.2}{\sqrt{12}} = 1.50$$

(b) To estimate with 90% confidence, we require the value of Z which includes 90% probability, i.e. excludes 5% in each tail. Thus $\phi(Z)$ or the CDF will be 0.95 to exclude 0.05 in the right-hand tail. To find this we must look in the body of the standard normal distribution table for 0.95 to determine the corresponding Z value. The closest we can get to it is 0.9495 or 0.9505 corresponding to $Z = 1.64$ and 1.65 respectively, so we estimate that $Z = 1.645$. To exclude 5%, or 0.05, in the left-hand tail, because the distribution is symmetrical, $Z = -1.645$. Since we are concerned with the mean of a sample, the relevant measure of variability (standard deviation) is the standard error of the mean, so that:

$$Z = \frac{\bar{x} - \mu}{\sigma/\sqrt{n}}$$

$$\therefore \quad \bar{x} = \mu + Z(\sigma/\sqrt{n})$$

$$= 14.1 \pm 1.645(5.2/\sqrt{12})$$

$$= 14.1 \pm 2.5$$

i.e. $11.6 < \bar{x} < 16.6$

Remember that when the number of degrees of freedom is very large, strictly infinity, the t-distribution becomes identical to the normal distribution, so as an alternative we can look at the t-distribution (Table B) at an infinite number of degrees of freedom. For a two-way significance test at 0.10, i.e. to exclude 10%, or to include 90%, we find 1.645. Such values are represented in some texts as the 'percentage points of the normal distribution'.

(c) We are unable to use the t-distribution at an infinite number of degrees of freedom to estimate the interquartile range because the appropriate value (excluding 25% in the tail) is not included in the table. We must, therefore, refer to the normal distribution (Table A) and seek a value of Z such that $\phi(Z) = 0.75$ to exclude 25% in the right-hand tail. We find that $\phi(0.67) = 0.7486$ and $\phi(0.68) = 0.7517$, so once again we can estimate that for $\phi(Z) = 0.75$ the required value of Z is 0.675. To exclude 25% in the left-hand tail, $Z = -0.675$.

Therefore $Z = \pm 0.675$ and, since in this case we are not concerned with the mean of a sample, the standard deviation is used.

$$Z = \frac{x - \mu}{\sigma}$$

$$x = \mu + Z(\sigma)$$

$$= 14.1 \pm 0.675(5.2)$$

$$= 14.1 \pm 3.5$$

thus the interquartile range is 10.6 to 17.6 mm.

Answer 5.4

(a) From the data:

$$\bar{x} = 7.39 \quad s = 1.059 \quad n = 30$$

Since this is a relatively large sample we may assume that the sample standard deviation is a reasonable estimation of the population value, thus the normal distribution may be used.

$$Z = \frac{\bar{x} - \mu}{\sigma/\sqrt{n}}$$

$$\therefore \quad \mu = \bar{x} - Z(\sigma/\sqrt{n})$$

$$= 7.39 \pm 1.96(1.059/\sqrt{30})$$

$$= 7.39 \pm 0.38$$

i.e. $7.01 < \mu < 7.77$

(b) (i)

$$Z = \frac{x - \mu}{\sigma}$$

$$= \frac{7.0 - 6.69}{1.22}$$

$$= 0.254$$

From Table A we find that $\phi(0.25) = 0.5987$, i.e. the probability that $Z < 0.25$ if the mean and standard deviation are 6.69 and 1.22 respectively is 0.5987. Thus the probability that $Z > 0.25$, or $x > 7.0$, is $(1 - 0.5987) = 0.4013$.

The effect of the third decimal place in the value of Z can be estimated by assuming that the difference between $\phi(0.25)$ and $\phi(0.26)$ is linear and if 0.4 of this difference is added to $\phi(0.25)$ we arrive at $\phi(0.254) = 0.6003$ so that the probability that $x > 7.0$ becomes $(1 - 0.6003) = 0.3997$, which, however, makes very little difference.

We would therefore conclude that 40.0% of the population would be expected to have a pinch grip strength greater than 7.0 kg.

(ii)

$$Z = \frac{x - \mu}{\rho}$$

$$= \frac{5.0 - 6.69}{1.22}$$

$$= -1.385$$

From Table A, taking the value midway between $+1.38$ and $+1.39$ we can estimate that $\phi(+1.385) = 0.9169$. Thus the probability that $Z > +1.385$ is $(1 - 0.9169) = 0.0831$, or, because the distribution is symmetrical, we can say that this is the same as the probability that $Z < -1.385$. Therefore the probability that the tip pinch grip strength (x) is less than 5.0 is 0.0831, so we would expect 8.3% of the population to be below this value.

(iii)

$$Z_1 = -0.566 \quad Z_2 = 1.074$$

From Table A, estimating the effect of the third decimal place:

$$P(Z < +0.566) = 0.7143 \quad P(Z < 1.074) = 0.8586$$

$$\therefore \quad P(Z > +0.566) = P(Z < -0.566) = (1 - 0.7143)$$
$$= 0.2857$$

$$\therefore \quad P(-0.566 < Z < 1.072) = 0.8586 - 0.2857$$
$$= 0.5729$$

Therefore we would expect 57.3% of the population to have a tip pinch strength of between 6.0 and 8.0 kg.

Answer 5.5

Firstly, we make the assumption that hip flexion range follows a normal distribution. We require the value of Z which will exclude 20% in the right-hand tail (22 subjects represent 20% of the total), i.e. that value for which ϕ, or the CDF, is 0.80. The closest we can get is 0.7995 when $Z = 0.84$, or 0.8023 when $Z = 0.85$, from which we can estimate that $Z = 0.842$.

In case this is not clear, the explanation is as follows:

(a) the difference between 0.7995 and 0.8023 is 0.0028;
(b) the difference between 0.7995 and 0.8000 (the required value) is 0.0005;
(c) 0.0005 as a fraction of the difference 0.0028 is 0.0005/ 0.0028 = 0.178 ≈ 0.2;
(d) therefore 0.2 of the third decimal place is added to $Z = 0.842$.

We can now write:

$$Z = \frac{x - \mu}{\sigma}$$

$$0.842 = \frac{140 - 125.2}{\sigma}$$

$$\therefore \quad \sigma = 17.6$$

Answers for Chapter 6

Answer 6.1

A two-sample one-way t-test is appropriate in this case.
The means and standard deviations of the samples are:

$$n_A = 10 \ df_A = 9 \quad \bar{x}_A = 13.6 \quad s_A = 12.18$$

$$n_B = 8 \ \ df_B = 7 \quad \bar{x}_B = 0.625 \quad s_B = 6.968$$

(a) The experimental hypothesis is that the mean of Group A is greater than the mean of Group B and the null hypothesis is that it is not, i.e.

$$H_0: \ \mu_A = \mu_B$$

$$H_1: \ \mu_A > \mu_B$$

Making the assumption that the two sample standard deviations are not significantly different, the value of the pooled estimate (s_p) and hence the value of t may now be calculated:

$$s_p = \sqrt{\frac{(n_A - 1)s_A^2 + (n_B - 1)s_B^2}{(n_A - 1) + (n_B - 1)}}$$

$$= \sqrt{\frac{9(12.18)^2 + 7(6.968)^2}{9 + 7}}$$

$$= 10.23$$

and

$$t_0(df = 16) = \frac{(\bar{x}_A - \bar{x}_B) - (\mu_A - \mu_B)}{s_P\sqrt{\dfrac{1}{n_A} + \dfrac{1}{n_B}}}$$

$$= \frac{(13.6 - 0.625) - 0}{10.23\sqrt{\dfrac{1}{10} + \dfrac{1}{8}}}$$

$$= 2.67$$

From the tables we can see that, at 16 degrees of freedom, the values of t with 1% and 0.5% in a single tail are 2.583 and 2.921, respectively. Remember that this means that there is a probability of 0.01 (or 1%) that, by random chance alone, if H_0 is true, t will exceed 2.583, and a probability of 0.005 (0.5%) that it will exceed 2.921. Therefore the probability that t will exceed 2.67, the calculated value in this case, lies between 0.005 and 0.01, i.e.

$$0.005 < P < 0.01$$

Thus the conclusion is that the difference is significant at the 1% level, i.e. there is a less than 1% probability that the observed difference has occurred by chance, and therefore the training is successful.

Alternatively, we may say that we draw this conclusion with 99% confidence.

(b) Group A: for the 98% confidence interval (compare Example 6.5) we require the values of t with 9 degrees of freedom, which contain a probability of 1% in each tail, i.e. $t = +2.821$.

The relevant calculation is therefore:

$$\mu_A = \bar{x}_A - t\left(\frac{s_A}{\sqrt{n_A}}\right)$$

$$= 13.6 + 2.821\left(\frac{12.2}{\sqrt{10}}\right)$$

$$= 13.6 \pm 10.9$$

which would be reported as:

$$2.7 < \mu_A < 24.5$$

and for Group B we require the tabulated value of t with 7 degrees of freedom, namely $t = \pm2.998$

$$\mu_B = 0.62 \pm 2.998\left(\frac{6.97}{\sqrt{8}}\right)$$

$$= 0.62 \pm 7.39$$

Therefore:

$$-6.8 < \mu_B < 8.0$$

Note that when the samples are considered separately, the number of degrees of freedom and the standard deviation appropriate to each is used.

(c) The 'random variable' is now the difference between the means (compare Equation 6.1) so that t becomes:

$$t = \frac{(\bar{x}_A - \bar{x}_B) - (\mu_A - \mu_B)}{SE_{(\bar{x}_A - \bar{x}_B)}}$$

Referring to Equations 6.3 and 6.4, for 95% confidence limits, the equation may be rearranged:

$$(\mu_A - \mu_B) = (\bar{x}_A - \bar{x}_B) \pm t_{0.025}(df = 16)s_P\sqrt{\frac{1}{10} + \frac{1}{8}}$$

where:

$$s_P = \sqrt{\frac{(n_A - 1)s_A^2 + (n_B - 1)s_B^2}{(n_A - 1) + (n_B - 1)}} = 10.23$$

substituting:

$$(\mu_A - \mu_B) = 12.97 \pm (2.120)(10.23)\sqrt{\frac{1}{10} + \frac{1}{8}}$$

$$= 12.97 \pm 10.29$$

so that:

$$2.7 < (\mu_A - \mu_B) < 23.3$$

Answer 6.2

The relevant hypotheses are:

$$H_0: \mu_A = \mu_B$$

$$H_1: \mu_A \neq \mu_B$$

If we assume that the standard deviations of the samples are not significantly different ($s_A = 36.6$ and $s_B = 33.9$) a pooled samples t-test is applied. This may be confirmed using an F-test (see Chapter 8) if desired. The pooled standard deviation (compare Equation 6.4) is given by:

$$s_P = \sqrt{\frac{(n_A - 1)s_A^2 + (n_B - 1)s_B^2}{(n_A - 1) + (n_B - 1)}}$$

$$= \sqrt{\frac{7(36.6)^2 + 5(33.9)^2}{7 + 5}}$$

$$= 35.5$$

and:

$$t = \frac{(\bar{x}_A - \bar{x}_B) - (\mu_A - \mu_B)}{s_P\sqrt{\dfrac{1}{n_A} + \dfrac{1}{n_B}}}$$

$$= \frac{(526.1 - 472.7) - 0}{35.5\sqrt{\dfrac{1}{8} + \dfrac{1}{6}}}$$

$$= 2.79$$

with 12 degrees of freedom, $(n-1)$ from each sample. Remember that, since the difference between the samples is arbitrarily positive or negative, it is convenient to take the positive option, thus:

$$0.01 < P < 0.02$$

for a two-way test. We would therefore reject the null hypothesis and conclude that the difference in the PEF of the two groups is significant at the 2% level.

Answer 6.3

In this test we are concerned with different individuals whose normal reaction times may well be quite different, thus the 'before' and 'after' times represent repeated measures so a paired sample or related t-test is appropriate. The mean and standard deviation of the differences are determined and t may be calculated by:

$$t_0 = \frac{\bar{d} - \mu_d}{s_d/\sqrt{n}} = \frac{0.018\,75 - 0}{0.017\,27/\sqrt{8}} = 3.07$$

i.e. for a one-way test:

$$0.005 < P < 0.01$$

The probability that the observed differences have occurred by chance is very small (less than 1%) so we reject the null hypothesis and conclude that the consumption of alcohol reduces the reaction time.

Answer 6.4

(a) A paired sample one-way t-test is appropriate for this problem:

$$t_0 = \frac{\bar{d} - \mu_d}{s_d/\sqrt{n}} = \frac{4.0 - 0}{4.472/\sqrt{10}} = 2.83$$

Remember to include the difference of zero (for subject H) when calculating the mean and standard deviation of the differences.

From the tables we find that:

$$0.005 < P < 0.01$$

i.e. the difference is highly significant.

(b) The above equation for t is rearranged:

$$\mu_d = \bar{d} - t\left(\frac{s_d}{\sqrt{10}}\right)$$

To include a probability of 95%, t takes the value (with 9 degrees of freedom) of ± 2.262. Thus we conclude that:

$$\mu_d = 4.0 \pm 3.2$$

$$0.8 < \mu_d < 7.2$$

Answer 6.5

(a) $\bar{x}_A = 56.50 \quad s_A = 5.717$

$\bar{x}_B = 59.20 \quad s_B = 6.296$

(b) The samples are independent and the relevant experimental hypotheses are:

$$H_0: \quad \mu_A = \mu_B$$
$$H_1: \quad \mu_A < \mu_B$$

i.e. a two sample one-way t-test is required.
   The pooled estimate of the standard deviation is given by:

$$s_p = \sqrt{\frac{19(5.717)^2 + 19(6.296)^2}{19 + 19}}$$

$$= 6.01$$

and

$$t_0(df = 38) = \frac{(59.20 - 56.50)}{6.01\sqrt{\dfrac{1}{20} + \dfrac{1}{20}}} = 1.42$$

From Table B we find that at 38 degrees of freedom:

$$0.05 < P < 0.10$$

i.e. there is rather more than a 5% probability that the observed difference has occurred by chance. The claim that method B is superior is, therefore, not supported.

(c) The values of t which include a probability of 95%, i.e. exclude 2.5% in each tail, are ± 2.093 at 19 degrees of freedom.

$$\mu_A = \bar{x}_A - t\left(\frac{s_A}{\sqrt{n_A}}\right)$$

$$= 56.50 \pm 2.093\left(\frac{5.717}{\sqrt{20}}\right)$$

$$= 56.5 \pm 2.7$$

i.e.

$$53.8 < \mu_A < 59.2$$

Similarly:

$$56.3 < \mu_B < 62.1$$

Answers for Chapter 7

Answer 7.1

$$\chi_0^2(\mathrm{df} = 4) = 8.41 \quad 0.05 < P < 0.10$$

There is a greater than 5% probability that the difference between the proportions has occurred by chance, so we would conclude that this is the case and that the responses are independent of the category of the respondent, i.e. there is insufficient evidence to reject the null hypothesis:

$$H_0: \; p_1 = p_2 = p_3$$

Answer 7.2

The expected values are shown in brackets:

		Age group			
		20–29	30–39	40–49	50–59
Number of visits	<3	5 (4.76)	14 (11.90)	12 (14.29)	9 (9.05)
	3–5	2 (2.02)	6 (5.06)	7 (6.07)	2 (3.85)
	>5	3 (3.21)	5 (8.04)	11 (9.64)	8 (6.11)

You will note that four of the 12 cells have expected frequencies less than 5, which is more than the acceptable 20%. The alternatives open to us are either to obtain more data by interviewing a larger number of people, or to combine some of the categories. If we assume that the former option is not possible, we must combine the first two groups to produce the following contingency table:

		Age group		
		20–39	40–49	50–59
Number of	<3	19 (16.67)	12 (14.29)	9 (9.05)
visits	3–5	8 (7.08)	7 (6.07)	2 (3.85)
	>5	8 (11.25)	11 (9.64)	8 (6.11)

We now have only a single cell with an expected frequency less than 5, which is acceptable.

$$\chi_0^2(\text{df} = 4) = 3.56$$

from the tables we find that $P > 0.20$. Thus we cannot reject the null hypothesis so we must conclude that there is not a significant difference between the frequency of visits and the age group of the patient.

We have, of course, lost some information because the sample size was rather small, i.e. the first two age groups covering 10 years each are now condensed into a single group covering 20 years.

Answer 7.3

We have a 2 × 2 contingency table with a single degree of freedom so the Yates correction is applied (see Equation 7.2). Remember that $|O - E|$ means that the 'modulus' of the difference between the observed and expected values, that is the positive value of the difference irrespective of the sign.

$$\chi_0^2(\text{df} = 1) = 2.87$$

From the tables we find:

$$0.05 < P < 0.10$$

The probability that the observed difference has occurred by chance is greater than 5%, the specified significance level. Thus there is insufficient evidence for us to reject the null hypothesis, so we must accept it and conclude that there is not a significant difference between the two treatments.

Answer 7.4

$$\chi^2(\text{df} = 4) = 10.36 \quad 0.025 < P < 0.05$$

The null hypothesis is therefore rejected and we conclude that the mental state is not independent of physical build.

Answer 7.5

(a)
$$\frac{9}{174} \times 100 = 5.2\% \quad \frac{5}{295} \times 100 = 1.7\%$$

Remember that percentages must never be used in a contingency table because the value of chi-square obtained is sensitive to sample sizes.

(b) In this case, the alternative hypothesis is that the proportions are unequal:

$$H_1 : p_1 \neq p_2$$

so we employ a non-directional or two-way test. This is the 'norm' for a chi-square test.

The contingency table:

	Premature	Normal	Total
Myopic	9 (5.19)	5 (8.81)	14
Normal	165 (168.81)	290 (286.19)	455
Total	174	295	469

Including the Yates correction:

$$\chi^2(df = 1) = 3.45$$

From the tables we find:

$$0.05 < P < 0.10$$

so we are unable to reject the null hypothesis and must conclude that there is no difference between the ratios in the two groups.

(c) To answer this question a directional test is employed. The alternative or experimental hypothesis in this case is:

$$H_1: \; p_{\text{Premature}} > p_{\text{Normal}}$$

where p represents the ratio myopic/normal sight.

We now find that:

$$0.025 < P < 0.05$$

Thus, at the 5% level of significance, we reject the null hypothesis in favour of the alternative and conclude that the ratio myopic/normal sight is greater in the case of premature births.

Remember that a directional test such as this is only possible in the case of a 2 × 2 chi-square test.

Answers for Chapter 8

Answer 8.1

(a)

	A	B	C	D	
	18	28	23	21	
	21	30	29	23	
	24	26	28	27	
	18	32	30	21	
	28	31	25	20	
Total	109	+ 147	+ 135	+ 112	= 503

The total sum of the squares (SST) and the sum of the squares of the columns (SSC) may now be calculated:

$$SST = \sum x^2 - \frac{G^2}{N}$$

$$= (18^2 + 21^2 + 24^2 + \cdots + 21^2 + 20^2) - \frac{503^2}{20}$$

$$= 13{,}013 - 12{,}650.45$$

$$= 362.55$$

$$SSC = \sum \frac{T_c^2}{n_r} - \frac{G^2}{N}$$

$$= \left(\frac{109^2}{5} + \frac{147^2}{5} + \frac{135^2}{5} + \frac{112^2}{5} \right) - \frac{503^2}{20}$$

$$= 12{,}851.8 - 12{,}650.45$$

$$= 201.35$$

and the sum of the squares of the error is obtained by subtraction:

$$SSE = SST - SSC$$

$$= 362.55 - 201.35$$

$$= 161.20$$

The ANOVA table may now be constructed:

Source of variation	SS	df	MS	F
Column means	201.35	3	67.12	6.66
Error	161.20	16	10.075	
Total	362.55	19		

The value of F obtained is highly significant:

$$P < 0.01$$

We therefore reject the null hypothesis in favour of the alternative and conclude that the means are not all equal.

(b) The probability of correctly rejecting the null hypothesis in all the t-tests becomes quite small. The number of t-tests that would be required to compare each sample with each of the others is given by the number of different ways of selecting x items from n, where in this case $x = 2$ and $n = 4$, i.e.

$$^nC_x = \frac{n!}{x!\,(n-x)!} = \frac{4!}{2!\,2!} = 6$$

(c) The least significant difference between the means is given by:

$$\text{LSD} = t_{0.025}(\text{df} = 16)s_w\sqrt{\frac{1}{n} + \frac{1}{n'}}$$

$$= 2.120\sqrt{10.075}\sqrt{\frac{1}{5} + \frac{1}{5}}$$

$$= 4.26$$

Arranging the means in order of magnitude:

$$\bar{x}_A \quad < \quad \bar{x}_D \quad < \quad \bar{x}_C \quad < \quad \bar{x}_B$$

$\bar{x}_A$		$\bar{x}_D$		$\bar{x}_C$		$\bar{x}_B$
21.8		22.4		27.0		29.4

| | 0.6 | | 4.6 | | 2.4 | |

i.e.

$$\underline{\mu_A \quad \mu_D} \qquad \underline{\mu_C \quad \mu_B}$$

Answer 8.2

A one-way ANOVA with repeated measures is the appropriate test. Remember that this amounts to a two-way ANOVA in which the sum of the squares of the rows is calculated so that it may be subtracted from the total sum of the squares in order to eliminate the variability between the subjects.

| | Week | | | | | Row total |
	1	2	3	4	5	
Mr A	25	21	20	18	20	104
Mr B	23	17	25	15	16	96
Mrs C	18	19	22	17	11	87
Miss D	27	20	23	24	19	113
Mr E	24	26	18	25	18	111
Mr F	25	27	17	17	16	102
Mrs G	26	20	20	19	19	104
Mrs H	20	26	20	17	18	101
Column total	188	176	165	152	137	818

$$\text{SST} = \sum x^2 - \frac{G^2}{N}$$

$$= (25^2 + 23^2 + 18^2 + \cdots + 19^2 + 18^2) - \frac{818^2}{40}$$

$$= 17,288 - 16,728.2$$

$$= 559.9$$

$$\text{SSC} = \Sigma \frac{T_c^2}{n_r} - \frac{G^2}{N}$$

$$= \left(\frac{188^2}{8} + \frac{176^2}{8} + \frac{165^2}{8} + \frac{152^2}{8} + \frac{137^2}{8} \right) - \frac{818^2}{40}$$

$$= 16,927.3 - 16,728.1$$

$$= 199.15$$

$$\text{SSR} = \sum \frac{T_r^2}{n_c} - \frac{G^2}{N}$$

$$= \left(\frac{104^2}{5} + \frac{96^2}{5} + \frac{87^2}{5} + \cdots + \frac{104^2}{5} + \frac{101^2}{5} \right) - \frac{818^2}{40}$$

$$= 16,822.4 - 16,728.1$$

$$= 94.3$$

$$SSE = SST - SSC - SSR$$
$$= 559.9 - 199.15 - 94.3$$
$$= 266.45$$

Source of variation	SS	df	MS	F(df = 4, 28)
Hours/week	199.15	4	49.79	49.79/9.52 = 5.23
Patient	94.30	7	13.47	
Error	266.45	28	9.52	
Total	559.95	39		

From Table D we can see that:

$$F_{0.01}(4, 28) = 4.07$$

Since the observed value is larger than this, there is a less than 1% probability that it has occurred by chance. Thus we would reject the null hypothesis and conclude that the average number and duration of headaches of the patients has changed as a result of therapy, i.e.

$$P < 0.01$$

Answer 8.3

The ANOVA table may be set up as follows:

Source of variation	SS	df	MS	F
Column means	1413.80	3	471.27	2.70
Error	4366.34	25	174.65	
Total	5780.14	28		

$$F_0(3, 25) = 2.70$$

From Table D we can see that:

$$F_{0.05}(3, 25) = 2.99$$

therefore $P > 0.05$ and the null hypothesis cannot be rejected, so we conclude that in this gymnasium the members from different professions do not have significantly different blood pressure.

Answer 8.4

This test requires a one-way analysis of variance. It is an extension of the independent sample t-test where there are more than two groups.

The sums of the squares may be calculated:

$$\text{SST} = \sum x^2 - \frac{G^2}{N} \quad \text{df} = (N - 1)$$

$$= 130,640 - \frac{(2026)^2}{32} = 2368.88$$

$$\text{SSC} = \sum \frac{T_k^2}{n_r} - \frac{G^2}{N} \quad \text{df} = (k - 1)$$

$$= \left(\frac{543^2 + 478^2 + 553^2 + 452^2}{8} \right) - \frac{(2026)^2}{32} = 909.63$$

The ANOVA table may now be set up:

Source of variation	Sum of the squares	DF	Mean square	$F(3, 28)$
Column means	909.63	3	303.21	$303.21/52.12 = 5.82$
Error	1,459.25	28	52.12	
Total	2,368.88	31		

From Table D it can be seen that, at 3 and 28 degrees of freedom, the observed value of $F(5.82)$ exceeds the critical value at 1% significance (4.57), i.e. $P < 0.01$, or there is a less than 1% probability that this value of F has occurred by chance, therefore the null hypothesis is rejected and we would conclude that the four methods of teaching are not equivalent.

In order to investigate further, the least significant difference (LSD) may be calculated at the 5% level. Remember that this is the lowest value of the difference between the means, based on the within-group, or pooled, estimate of the standard deviation, which is significant at the 5% level. The value of t employed is at the number of degrees of freedom corresponding to the error variance, in this case.

$$t_{0.025} = \frac{(\bar{x} - \bar{x}')}{s_w \sqrt{\frac{1}{8} + \frac{1}{8}}}$$

$$\text{or} \quad (\bar{x} - \bar{x}') = \text{LSD} = t_{0.025} s_w \sqrt{\frac{1}{8} + \frac{1}{8}}$$

$$= (2.048)\sqrt{52.12}(0.5)$$

$$= 7.39$$

where $(\bar{x} - \bar{x}')$ is the least significant difference (LSD) at the 5% level. Note that s_w, the within-group standard deviation, is the standard deviation of the error, i.e. the square root of the mean sum of the squares of the error.

Placing the sample means in order of magnitude we find:

	$\bar{x}_D$	<	$\bar{x}_B$	<	$\bar{x}_A$	<	$\bar{x}_C$
	56.50		59.75		67.88		69.13

Difference:	3.25		8.13		1.25

The differences between the means of samples D and B, and also between samples A and C are less than the least significant difference (7.39), but the pairs, differing by at least 8.13, are significantly different from each other.

This result may be expressed as follows:

$$\underline{\mu_D \quad \mu_B} \qquad \underline{\mu_A \quad \mu_C}$$

Answer 8.5

(a) This problem requires a straightforward one-way analysis of variance and after calculating the sums of the squares the following table may be constructed:

Source of variation	SS	DF	MS	$F(df = 3, 28)$
Column means	536.13	3	178.7	$178.7/41.4 = 4.32$
Error	1,159.7	28	41.4	
Total	1,659.9	31		

Consulting Table D shows that:

$$0.01 < P < 0.025$$

Therefore the null hypothesis is rejected and we conclude that at the 5% level of significance, the means are not all equal.

(b) To calculate the least significant difference, we require the value of t at 28 degrees of freedom which excludes 2.5% in each tail of the distribution. This is the 'protected t' with the number of degrees of freedom corresponding to the error term. The appropriate standard deviation is the pooled estimate from the 'error variance', namely $s_p = \sqrt{(41.4)} = 6.43$.

The least significant difference (LSD) may now be calculated:

$$t_{0.025}(df = 28) = \frac{LSD}{s_P\sqrt{\frac{1}{8}+\frac{1}{8}}}$$

$$LSD = t_{0.025}(df = 28)s_P\sqrt{\frac{1}{8}+\frac{1}{8}}$$

$$= (2.048)(6.43)\sqrt{\frac{1}{8}+\frac{1}{8}}$$

$$= 6.58$$

Placing the means in order we find:

$\bar{x}_D$	$<$	$\bar{x}_C$	$<$	$\bar{x}_A$	$<$	$\bar{x}_B$
46.75		54.38		54.75		57.88

Difference:	7.63	0.37	3.13

We can see that the difference between the means of samples D and C is significant, but C, A and B are not significantly different from each other. We may therefore write:

$$\mu_D \qquad \mu_C \quad \mu_A \quad \mu_B$$

Answer 8.6

This problem requires, in each case, a one-way analysis of variance with repeated measures, which is, effectively, a two-way analysis of variance, where the variability between subjects is eliminated. The variability between subjects may well be very significant and must, therefore, be eliminated so that variability between angles may be determined.

Firstly, for the dominant leg, the various sums of the squares may be calculated and the following table set up:

Source of variation	Sum of the squares	DF	Mean square	F
Subjects	297.636	10	29.76	12.45
Angles	5.515	2	2.76	1.15
Error	47.818	20	2.39	
Total	350.970	32		

For the variability between angles $F(2, 20) = 1.15$.

From the tables for the F-distribution (Table D) we can see that

$$F_{0.05}(2, 20) = 3.49:$$

Remember that this means that, if the null hypothesis is true and there is no difference between the strengths at different angles, F may take a value as large as 3.49, by chance alone, with a probability of 0.05, or 5%. Thus the observed value, 1.15, may occur by chance with a probability greater than 5% so there is insufficient evidence to reject the null hypothesis and we would therefore conclude that the strengths of the quadriceps measured at the three different angles are not significantly different at the 5% level, which may be represented:

$$P > 0.05$$

Since 1.15 is a good deal less than the critical value of 3.49, we would conclude that P is a good deal larger than 0.05. With a fairly limited set of tables, it is not possible to establish this, but using the computer package MINITAB it can be demonstrated that $P = 0.337$.

As a matter of interest, the critical value which is relevant to the variability between subjects, i.e. at 10 and 20 degrees of freedom, can be estimated from Table D (since only $F(9, 20)$ and $F(12, 20)$ are quoted) to be 3.38 at 1%, i.e. at $P = 0.01$. The observed value of 12.45 is well in excess of this so that $P \ll 0.01$, in fact MINITAB tells us that $P < 0.0001$. Remember that this means that the probability that the observed differences between subjects having arisen by chance alone is exceedingly small, in fact virtually zero, which is not surprising.

An exactly similar procedure is followed for the non-dominant leg resulting in the ANOVA table:

Source of variation	Sum of the squares	DF	Mean square	F
Subjects	203.576	10	20.358	12.49
Angles	8.061	2	4.030	2.47
Error	32.606	20	1.630	
Total	244.242	33		

As before, we find that $P > 0.05$, i.e. the differences are not significant.

Answer 8.7

Calculating the average for the dominant and non-dominant legs and the difference for each subject results in the following:

Average dominant leg	Average non-dominant leg	Difference
13.333	15.000	−1.667
22.667	19.667	3.000
13.667	12.000	1.667
15.667	14.333	1.333
17.000	16.000	1.000
16.667	14.667	2.000
16.000	12.333	3.667
14.333	13.667	0.667
13.000	13.667	−0.667
13.333	15.333	−2.000
20.667	20.000	0.667

(a) **Paired sample t-test**

In this test, the null hypothesis is that the average difference (column 3 above) is zero. The mean and standard deviation of the difference are 0.879 and 1.778, respectively.

$$t = \frac{\bar{d} - \mu_d}{s_d/\sqrt{n}} \quad \text{where } \mu_d = \text{zero}$$

$$= \frac{0.879}{1.778/\sqrt{11}}$$

$$= 1.64 \quad (df = 10)$$

From Table B, it can be seen that for a non-directional test at 10 degrees of freedom:

$$0.10 < P < 0.20$$

i.e. the null hypothesis is accepted so we would conclude that there is no significant difference between the two samples.

(b) **Analysis of variance—one way with repeated measures**
The various sums of the squares are calculated in the normal manner and the ANOVA table set up as follows:

Source of variation	Sum of the squares	DF	Mean square	F
Subjects	151.263	10	15.126	
Leg (D/ND)	4.247	1	4.247	2.69
Error	15.808	10	1.581	
Total	171.318	21		

From Table D we find that:

$$F_{0.05}(1, 10) = 4.96$$

and, since

$$F(\text{observed}) < 4.96$$

we conclude that:

$$P > 0.05$$

If a computer package such as MINITAB is available, the exact value of P may be obtained and will be found to be 0.132 in both of the above exercises.

Answers for Chapter 9

Answer 9.1

A Mann–Whitney test is performed because there is no reason to believe that these data follow a normal distribution. The appropriate hypotheses are:

$$H_0: \ \mu_1 = \mu_2$$
$$H_1: \ \mu_1 \neq \mu_2$$

and from the data:

$$n_1 = 7 \qquad\qquad n_2 = 9$$
$$W_1 = 45 \qquad\qquad W_2 = 91$$
$$U_1 = W_1 - \frac{n_1(n_1 + 1)}{2} \qquad U_2 = W_2 - \frac{n_2(n_2 + 1)}{2}$$
$$= 17 \qquad\qquad\qquad = 46$$

For samples sized 7 and 9, it can be seen from Table E that the critical value for a two-way test, at the 10% level of significance, is 15. If the smaller value of U is equal to or less than the critical value, the difference between the means of the two groups is significant at that level.

In this case:

$$P > 0.10$$

i.e. there is insufficient evidence to reject the null hypothesis at the 10%, and also, of course, also at the 5% level of significance. We therefore would conclude that there is not a significant difference in the difficulty in speech experienced by the two groups.

Answer 9.2

A Mann–Whitney U test is appropriate. The claim is that Method I is superior to Method II so the appropriate hypotheses are:

$$H_0: \ \mu_1 = \mu_2$$

$$H_1: \ \mu_1 < \mu_2$$

i.e. a one-way, or directional test is performed and U_1 only needs be calculated:

$$n_1 = 6$$

$$W_1 = 34$$

$$U_1 = W_1 - \frac{n_1(n_1 + 1)}{2}$$

$$= 13$$

Consulting Table E, it can be seen that for a one-way test for samples of size 6 and 9, the critical value of U at the 5% level of significance is 12. Since the observed value, 13, is larger than this, we cannot reject the null hypothesis, although it is rather close, and we must conclude that there is not a significant difference between the methods at the 5% level, i.e.

$$P > 0.05$$

Answer 9.3

The hypotheses are, of course, the same as in the Answer 9.2, and U_1 is calculated:

$$n_1 = 12$$

$$W_1 = 130$$

$$U_1 = W_1 - \frac{n_1(n_1 + 1)}{2}$$

$$= 52$$

Referring to Table E once again shows that, for sample sizes 12 and 18, the critical value at the 1% level is 53. Thus the observed value of 52 is significant (just) at that level. A quite different conclusion from that reached in Exercise 9.2 as a result of the samples being larger, i.e.

$$P < 0.01$$

We would therefore conclude that Method I is superior to Method II.

Answer 9.4

When the data are combined and ranked, the following table may be set up.

Group A		Group B		Group C	
Score	Rank	Score	Rank	Score	Rank
4	2.5	4	2.5	5	8.5
4	2.5	5	8.5	5	8.5
4	2.5	5	8.5	5	8.5
5	8.5	6	16	6	16
5	8.5	6	16	6	16
5	8.5	7	21	7	21
6	16	8	26.5	8	26.5
6	16	8	26.5	8	26.5
6	16	9	32	8	26.5
7	21	9	32	8	26.5
8	26.5	10	35	9	32
8	26.5	10	35	10	35
Rank sum = 155		259.5		251.5	

The Kruskal–Wallis statistic is calculated:

$$H = \frac{12}{N(N+1)} \sum \frac{R^2}{n} - 3(N+1)$$

$$= \frac{12}{(36)(37)} \left(\frac{155^2}{12} + \frac{259.5^2}{12} + \frac{251.5^2}{12} \right) - 3(37)$$

$$= 5.08$$

This value is tested for significance against χ^2 at 2 degrees of freedom, i.e. $(k-1)$, whereupon we conclude that:

$$0.05 < P < 0.10$$

There is, therefore, insufficient evidence to reject the null hypothesis. We conclude that there is no difference between the assessments.

Answer 9.5

A non-parametric repeated measures test is appropriate here, i.e. the Wilcoxon signed-rank test. The differences between the scores are calculated and ranked, disregarding the sign and omitting those for which the differences are zero. Remember that differences which are equal are assigned an average rank.

Patient	Before viewing	After viewing	Difference	Rank of difference ignoring the sign
1	2	1	-1	2 $(-)$
2	2	0	-2	4 $(-)$
3	3	0	-3	5.5 $(-)$
4	0	0	omit	
5	3	3	omit	
6	1	1	omit	
7	1	2	$+1$	2 $(+)$
8	3	0	-3	5.5 $(-)$
9	1	0	-1	2 $(-)$
10	0	0	omit	

$$W_- = 2 + 4 + 5.5 + 5.5 + 2 = 19$$
$$W_+ = 2$$

The relevant hypotheses are (A = after viewing and B = before viewing):

$$H_0 : \mu_A = \mu_B$$

$$H_1 : \mu_A < \mu_B$$

The smaller of the two values for the rank sums is compared for significance with Table F. For $n = 6$ (remember that the observations where the difference is zero are not counted) for a one-way test the value of 2 is significant at $P = 0.05$. There is sufficient evidence for us to reject the null hypothesis in favour of the experimental hypothesis so we conclude that viewing the video reduces anxiety in the patients.

Answer 9.6

This problem requires a non-parametric analysis of variance with repeated measures, i.e. a Friedman test. The score for each tutor under the three conditions (methods of presentation) are ranked and the sum of the ranks for each condition is obtained.

	A		B		C	
Tutor	Score	Rank	Score	Rank	Score	Rank
1	15	2	10	1	17	3
2	12	2	11	1	19	3
3	17	2.5	13	1	17	2.5
4	14	2	10	1	15	3
5	10	1	12	3	11	2
Rank sum		9.5		7		13.5

The Friedman statistic may now be calculated for $n = 5$ and $k = 3$:

$$M = \frac{12}{nk(k+1)} \sum R^2 - 3n(k+1)$$

$$= \frac{12}{(5)(3)(4)} (9.5^2 + 7.0^2 + 13.5^2) - 3(5)(4)$$

$$= 4.30$$

From Table J we find that for $k = 3$ and $n = 5$ the calculated value of M, 4.30, is smaller than the value at $P = 0.10$, therefore it is not significant. We conclude, therefore, that the audiences do not perceive a significant difference between the three methods of presentation.

Index